Return to Eden
An Herbal Medicine Field Guide

JUDITH M. ERVINE, SRN

With contributions by

ANGELA KATSIRI

Registered Herbal Practitioner

Sketches by Ryan Ervine

Copyright © 2011 Judith M. Ervine

All rights reserved.

ISBN – 10: 1466364297
ISBN-13: 978-1466364295

DEDICATION

Firstly I dedicate this book to Father God. My life has been a journey. Thank you for patiently walking next to me, for often carrying me, leading me and showing me the way forward.

Secondly I dedicate this book to my family – My husband Rory and our sons, Sean, Craig and Ryan. For putting up with me over the years and forgiving me for making you eat all those horrible tasting plants when you were ill. I thank God for you all every day.

Thirdly to my mother – Betty Bromley, who knew my dream and bought me my first herbal book. She also helped me develop my gift from the Father for art.

CONTENTS

Acknowledgements	13
Introduction	15
Judy's Testimony	19
Angela's Testimony	25
References and Reading List	31
Eden Herbal Medical Clinic History	33
Herbs ARE Medicine Disclaimer	37
Herbal Remedies and Recipes	39
Abscesses	40
AIDS	41
Anaemia	42
Antibiotic Ointment	43
Anti-Itch Ointment	44
Antiseptic Wash	45
Arthritis Regime	46
Asthma	48
Asthma Regime	49

Asthma Syrup	50
Bilharzia	51
Breast Lumps and Pain	53
Bronchitis, Flu, Common Cold	54
Burns	57
Camphor Rub	58
Cancer	59
Cancer Syrup	61
Candida	62
Candida Mouthwash	63
Cayenne Pepper Ointment	64
Chicken Pox	65
Chicken Pox Lotion	66
Conjunctivitis	67
Constipation	68
Cough Mixture – Adult	69
Cough Mixture – Children	70
Cough Mixture – Garlic Remedy	71
Cough Mixture – Ginger & Sugar	72

Cough Mixture – Lemon & Ginger	73
Cough Mixture – Tickle	74
Diabetes	75
Diarrhea	76
Diarrhea Mixture	77
Diarrhea Syrup	78
Diuretic	79
Ear Infections	80
Ear Drops – Yarrow Garlic	81
Ear Drops – Tea Tree	82
Eczema	83
Embrocation	85
Epilepsy Treatment	86
Eye Drops	87
Fever	88
Fungal Infections	90
Gastritis	91
Hemorrhoid's	92
Hemorrhoid Soothing Bath Oil	94

Headache	95
Heart Disease	96
Heart Care	98
Heart Stress Relieving Tea	99
Herbal Oils	100
Herbal Vinegars	102
Herpes	103
Insect Bites and Stings	104
Insect Repellant	105
Insomnia	107
Jaundice	108
Kidney Disease and Urinary Tract Infections	109
Lactation and Weaning	111
Malaria	112
Menstruation Problems	113
Migraine Headache	114
Nausea	115
Oedema	116
Poisoning	117

Scabies	118
Sexually Transmitted Diseases	119
Strokes	121
Toothache	123
Toothpaste	125
Tuberculosis	126
UTI regime	127
Venereal Disease	129
Vomiting	130
Warts and Verrucas	131
Wart Ointment	132
Worms	133
Worm Treatment	134
Wound Care	135
Yarrow Cream	136
Herbs and Their Uses	137
Aloe Vera *(Aloe vera/forex)*	138
Basil *(Ocimum basilicum)*	139
Blackjack *(Bidens pilosa)*	140

Bulbinella *(Bulbine frutescens)* — 141

Chickweed *(Stellaria media)* — 142

Dill *(Anethum graveolens)* — 143

Feverfew *(Chrysanthemum parthenium)* — 144

Garlic *(Allium sativum)* — 146

Ginger *(Zingiber officinalis)* — 148

Lavender *(Lavandula spica)* — 149

Lemon Grass *(Cymbopogan citrates)* — 150

Marjoram or Oregano *(Origanum vulgare)* — 152

Mint *(Mentha)* — 153

Moringa *(Moringa olefera)* — 154

Nasturtium *(Tropaeolum majus)* — 156

Neem *(Azadirachta indica)* — 158

Parsley *(Petroselinum crispum)* — 162

Rocket or Arugula *(Eruca vesicaria)* — 163

Rosemary *(Rosmarinus officinalis)* — 164

Rue *(Ruta graveolens)* — 165

Soapwort *(Saponaria officinalis)* — 167

Sour Fig *(Carpobrotus edulis)* — 168

Sweet Violet *(Viola odorata)*	169
Sweet Wormwood *(Artemesia afra)*	170
Tansy *(Tanacetum vulgare)*	172
Tea Tree *(Melaleuca alternifolia)*	173
Thyme *(Thymus vulgaris)*	175
Yarrow *(Achillea millefolium)*	176
Clinic Internships and Training in Herbal Medicine	179
Our Basic Needs	181
Our Dream	183
About the Author	185

ACKNOWLEDGMENTS

I hope and believe that many people will benefit from this book, whether locally in Zimbabwe or in other countries.

However there are many credits due:

Firstly a big thank-you to our Father who has made this book possible. Without Him, none of this would have happened and the journey I have taken would have been very different.

Kevin & Susan Fry, who have worked hard and taken the time to help put this book together and have encouraged me all the way.

Gordon & Dawn Aylward who kept on pestering me about getting the pictures done and the information down. Thank you for the belief in me that I could do it.

Angela and the Clinic team. You have been such an inspiration to me as well as to the community. You have done amazing things and given of yourselves to do it.

Closer to home, my husband Rory who has always encouraged me to get the book done and whom has helped me fulfil a dream and to keep looking up to the Lord and forward to hope for the future.

Our three sons – Sean, Craig & Ryan, who have often been at the receiving end of new herbal treatments. Thank you for believing in me and encouraging me. Ryan for the sketches he did. They are great.

INTRODUCTION & TESTIMONIES

When we talk about herbs, what do we mean?

The classical botanical definition of an herb is a soft stemmed plant that is an annual not a perennial. So what about the roots, bark, and fungi that are used for herbal medicine?

Anything that grows is really an herb as anything that God has created to grow whether vegetable, flower, weeds, trees, shrubs, wild plant, fungi or even mistletoe has some medicinal value. However we still don't know all their values yet. Many modern medicines today have their roots in plants e.g. Aspirin and Digitalis to name a few. Even the Malaria drug treatment at home today is partly derived from a plant. (Artemisia Anamed)

We have not managed to cover every herb that we use as many of these are from the wild and would not be recognised but we have tried to include the common ones.

What we are really showing you in this book are the recipes and plants that we use at Eden Clinic to help the people at Eden including the children and the people in the community.

Safety for herbal users

Herbal treatments are accumulative and therefore usually need to be taken over a period of time. Also don't be fooled by the fact that it is just a plant and so therefore not toxic or dangerous. Taking herbal medicine is not risk free although it is often safer than using conventional medicine because the herbs are maybe not as strong.

Some plants can be toxic in the wrong doses and we have added warnings to some of the plants that we work with because of this.

Identify correctly

If you are picking herbs in the wild, please make sure that you are absolutely sure about the herb that you are using. If there is any doubt in your mind about this then **DON'T** use it. Taking the wrong herb could be disastrous if it is a poisonous plant.

Herbs to avoid in pregnancy:

Feverfew

Rue

Wormwood

Tansy

Parsley – Eat only a little

Mints – Eat only a little

St John's Wort

Comfrey

Garlic

Side Effects:

People who use herbs may develop allergic reactions to some herbs. Signs like rashes and itchiness. Some people may even have a severe reaction and go into shock so please be cautious.

Interactions:

Pharmaceutical drugs and herbs can sometimes interact badly with each other. There can also be bad interactions between herbs when combinations of herbs are used.

For example Aspirin is a blood thinner but so is Vitamin E and Garlic to a certain degree. So please consult your doctor about using herbal medicine if you are on prescription drugs through your doctor.

We thank God for the miracles that He works in this small clinic which is only one room at the moment. But nothing is too small for the Lord and He is still a God of miracles today.

We pray that you will find this book interesting but also beneficial and also pray that one day you might be able to come out and see the clinic for yourself.

To Him is the glory!

Blessings!

Judy

Does it not make Sense

That God in His Sovereignty

Would create EVERYTHING

We would need

To Live well

On this earth?

Judy's Testimony

Actually I had not planned to do nursing originally. I had planned to be a vet because I love animals so much but my father had died when I was eight years old and although my mum had remarried, there was not enough money for seven years of training for a vetinary degree at that time. Nursing was the only other option because you were paid as you trained and there was no outlay.

I left school at the age of 18 years after completing my Cambridge 0 levels. I wanted to stay on to do Matric (South African M level) and A levels but my parents could not cope with the financial side. I went straight to the Andrew Fleming Hospital in Harare. It was the best hospital in southern Africa at that time. My training took three years and I remember at the start it felt like three years was a lifetime but it certainly went quickly. The university wing of the hospital was opened while I was there as a training ground for the university and we saw things that were amazing. I also saw that the rural people did not just believe in the western medicine but also in the herbal treatments and I would see the relatives coming into the wards with their packets of herbs to treat their relatives. I think that was when my first interest in herbal medicine was born. Also seeing the faith that people had put into the little packet of herbs was amazing.

To start with I struggled to cope with having to nurse people. I was an extremely shy person in those days and struggled to have conversations with people. (probably the reason why I wanted to work with animals instead of people) But gradually over the following months I began to really enjoy it and found my "niche" Some areas I didn't enjoy – Theatre being one, as there was no contact with people. I loved the old people wards and found older people very interesting. My grandmother was 97yrs and I used to love spending time with her and hearing about the "good old days". The children's wards I found really hard to cope with emotionally as the cases were so sad and often there was no hope. My nursing was during the bush war time so working in casualty

I had to deal with many war injuries. At that time I was engaged and Rory who was involved in the police force, was also in the middle of the war, it was an emotional time. I kept expecting a phone call but thank the Lord there was nothing serious.

My training finished in May 1980 and I was married the same year in July,. the year Zimbabwe got independence and changed from Rhodesia to Zimbabwe.

My husband Rory and I actually knew each other since junior school as we went to the same school together and our families had known each other for a long long time. He had been in the police force and now was working with his father on the family farm in the north of the country.

After we were married I joined him on the farm and then moved to Doma in 1982 where we farmed until 2001. I had a small clinic for the employees on the farm and was reading a lot about herbs and herbal medicine. I was also interested in the local bush herbs and tried to find out more knowledge about them from different sources, especially the older African people.

We have three boys – Sean born 1982, Craig born 1985 and Ryan born 1988. To bring the boys up on the farm was an amazing priviledge. They loved being outdoors in the bush and having different adventures camping and shooting. They always look back on their upbringing as a joy and it has given them a grounding that Africa is home. They still get very homesick when away from Zimbabwe.

We are also a sporting family so all three boys have made their careers in sport – Cricket. Sean now plays for Hampshire in the UK. Craig is playing nationally for Zimbabwe and Ryan is playing for the local franchise in Zimbabwe in the summer and has been playing for a club, Lisben, in Ireland in the UK summer.

We farmed in a remote farm in Doma as tobacco farmers but in 1993 the Lord really convicted us about the fact that growing a crop that was so unhealthy to the body was not what He wanted us to do. We knew that the money was in the tobacco and that if we gave it up we would probably not make it as farmers. This was the first time there were murmurings about the land seizure and our farm was one of the first names to come up. We gave up tobacco and had to sell the farm in 1995. The farm was also a game ranch and was bought by Safari Operators who asked us to stay on and manage the game operation. God knew that we were not ready to move. I was devastated. All our dreams had gone up in smoke. I remember arguing with the Lord and bargaining with him about the fact that we had done what He wanted and given up the Tobacco crop, so why had He not blessed the farm. We had even at one time wanted to start an orphanage there and to train the kids coming through in the different areas. The farm was called Eben farm. But the Lord never leaves us nor forsakes us and He had a plan that was better. It's a good thing we cannot see too far down the road.

In 2001, Kevin & Susan Fry asked us to come and work at Eden to do the farming and the medical side. We took the time to pray about it knowing in our hearts that we were still meant to stay in Zimbabwe and work with the people but didn't know where. We felt at peace about the decision to work at Eden and so moved across to a manager's cottage on the next door farm.

I myself was worried about how I was going to cope. I was angry at what had been done to people and what everyone had gone through. My mother had had a bleeding ulcer from when we had had to airlift out when they were trashing houses and she had died from a complication of pneumonia from that. Rory, my husband had spent time in jail because he was the "owner" of the farm although it had been sold by then and we were only managers. How on earth was I now going to go and look after African kids from the very same people who had destroyed so much?

But God is faithful and he changed me slowly but surely.

After being at Eden for a couple of weeks a family came for help carrying a child who was badly dehydrated and sick. I asked the father where they had come from. They said Eben (the farm that had been ours). I was furious and gave him a piece of my mind. But God tapped me on the shoulder and said look at the child. I will deal with the father but I need you to help the child. That was the turning point for me. It did not matter what people had done. That was God's problem. Mine was to help the children.

The herbal clinic hadn't been something that was planned. It was something that grew out of a need in the Doma area when the clinics were empty and people were suffering so much. An African lady had an abscess on her hand from reaping her corn and her father had approached my husband to ask for assistance with transport to the local hospital which is 25km away. He suggested that maybe she could see me as I am a state registered nurse and that I knew something about herbs. We did manage to treat her hand with herbs and it healed. She was our first patient and so from that day onwards word went around and we started to get people arriving with seriously infected wounds and different diseases, asking for help.

We first started under a tree and then moved to what used to be a chicken house. A crew from Goshen came and put up a one roomed building for us which has been great and up to date we have now had 21 000 people through the doors.

Why herbal medicine in this day and age where you can buy any tablet you need from a pharmacy. The main challenge we face out in Doma is that people don't have a dollar to spare for medicines. To spend a dollar on tablets for your child means you miss a meal that day. Also there are so many counterfeit drugs coming onto the market now, we have to ask ourselves the question – what is safe and what is not safe anymore. Herbal medicine has no additives that can cause allergies. It is natural, how God intended it to be. We run the clinic as a free clinic so that we can reach the people that need help. The children and the old and destitute. God our father has given us a pharmacy right outside out windows. We need to use it to the best of our ability.

At the clinic we work as a team. I am registered under the Traditional Medicine Association of Zimbabwe as a traditional healer. When I was registered they asked me which spirit I used for healing. I said the "Holy Spirit".

Angela is also registered as an herbal healer because of her time with the Catholic Herbal Structure. Laurence is a young man who I have trained up to do the dressings, lancing wounds and doing home visits. He is amazing and is really good at what he does. He reads a lot of medical books and one day we will try and get him into different medical training facilities to further his education. He is scrupulous in his cleanliness when dealing with some of the most awful cases that come in. We also have Joyce and Edzai who hand out the different herbs and give instructions on the treatments and how to take them. Elliot who is our village father is also the counsellor at the clinic. He also does the paper work for each patient. Everyone is registered through the clinic and everyone assists when collecting and processing the herbs.

Helping the elderly who are destitute and the children with malnutrition has also become a passion. It's amazing how God works because he will let you know when a person has come through the door that needs more than just a visit to the clinic and wants me to dig a little deeper. He does not lay that on my heart for everyone but just for a few at a time. We have had a few children placed at Eden Children's Village through the clinic as emergencies.

We also are here to serve people and the one way we serve is to speak to them about spiritual matters. The African culture is involved in a lot of cults and superstitions. From involvement with the different cults they come to the clinic wearing talismans around their arms, legs and waists. Especially the children. We speak to them about the fact that by wearing the strings they are putting their faith in the string instead of Jesus Christ. We actually refuse to treat them if they don't remove the strings as we tell them that here at the Eden Clinic our faith is in Jesus and not a piece of string. People will usually remove them. We burn them afterwards.

To start with when I saw local people I still thought about where they had come from and what they had done, but God has taken me even further than that. Now I just see people who are in need both physically and spiritually. We are God's servants and need to be servants to others. God is doing miracles today and we see them every day in what we all do whether it's in the clinic or in the school or in the farm.

We also train people from different areas in the country. At the moment we have six people coming from Harare to be trained. We do one week to start with and give them the basics then each week that they come we will get them more involved. They have so much to learn that we cannot tell it all in one week and they cannot absorb it all in one week either.

We have also had health workers form the different areas coming to learn about basic medicine, but this is difficult to follow up. One day hopefully when we have the mobile clinic up and running we will start a program of training health workers in their villages to help them become self sustainable while we follow up and advise them.

We don't know what the future holds but we do know that God holds our future. We do not take that journey alone. Thank the Lord, He walks beside us.

Angela's Testimony

My husband died in February 2001. I am a mother of four children -- A set of twins (boy and a girl) a daughter and a son.

At the time that my husband died he had been diagnosed with HIV/AIDS. I was very frustrated with my in-laws, as they refused to look after my husband while he was suffering but they wanted to take everything that he had and leave us destitute. I had been doing a lot of work through the Catholic Herbal Structure with Home Based Care in the community for six years so I could cope with the nursing of my husband but it was a difficult time emotionally for me. I felt that I had to close myself off emotionally to what was wrong with me and concentrate on my husband. It was my duty and I needed to be strong. I had some savings put by for the children's schooling but without the relatives help I had to use that for the care of my husband.

When I was diagnosed with HIV/AIDS, it did not come as a shock to me. Probably because I had been working closely with HIV/AIDS patients for the last six years and I knew deep inside that I had many of the same symptoms. What was frustrating was that my husband's family wanted me to release the children into their care as they said I was not going to live very long. I weighed 37kg (75lbs) at this stage. I refused and was adamant that I would live to take care of my own children.

I went to the Catholic Church which is where I worship, as they were starting an herbal structure workshop and also were starting a local support group for people in Chinhoyi town who were HIV/AIDS positive, so that they could help each other. I was already involved with them through their Home based Care program which I had been working in for 6 years. Through this program they were working in the community with people who had HIV/AIDS and also working with the relatives of people with HIV/AIDS and showing them how to look after their loved ones. They taught people how to bathe their sick ones, what nutritious food to give them, how to keep them comfortable when they were in pain and how to look after wounds and to dispose of bodily waste and clean the linen without contaminating themselves.

People did not know enough about the HIV/AIDS disease and there was a lot of superstition and ignorance involved. They found that people would hose their relatives down in the garden with a hose pipe and wash them with a grass broom because they did not want to get too close to them. When they visited some of the families they were told that the person who was sick was not there and they would hear someone calling weakly from inside the house to gain attention. People were being starved to death and living in the most appalling conditions. It was very depressing sometimes, but also rewarding when people listened to what they were taught and put it into practice and they saw families joining together to help loved ones.

However, I still had the problem as a new widow on how she was to get my children through school. I had the twins left to do schooling. I managed to raise enough capitol from the surrounding farms in Chinhoyi by working there and gleaning the maize and soya beans from their fields. I managed to start a small business of buying and selling in 2002 and the Catholic Herbal Structure group managed to help me with school fees for one child. I managed to pay for my second child to go to school. I also managed to buy a knitting machine so did knitting as part of my business. It was a very difficult time. I had to hold onto the Lord with all my strength and believe and stand on the word of God. The Lord was my only hope.

Through the herbal Structure Workshop I learnt about herbal identification, processing, ointment making and different remedies. I also started using the herbal remedies myself and my weight slowly crept up to 60kg (132lbs). I continued to work with the Home Based Care group in Chinhoyi as I have a real heart for the people. I felt I needed to be there for people and to give people with HIV/AIDS hope for the future and a hope in the Lord.

In the year 2004 I heard about the Eden Herbal Clinic that we were starting and thought she would like to be part of what Eden was doing. I came to see Judy and started working straight away. We see many HIV/AIDS patients and because I am positive I have been able to relate to people about their disease. I am an example of how a person can live with the HIV/AIDS virus and still be healthy.

There are four things that I have been very careful about with my health. I have cut right back on sugar and sugared drinks and foods, I take a mixture of ginger and garlic every morning, along with other herbs. I am very conscientious about my hygiene and I have a nutritious and balanced diet.

I chose not to go onto the anti-retroviral drugs or prophylaxis antibiotic drugs. This is not for everyone, but it has worked for me.

We see patients every second day and yet I have the most amazing resistance to cold and flu viruses that normally I would pick up from patients because we work out of a one room building.

In 2008 I had a retest and still tested positive for HIV. I also had my CD4 count done and it was 298 which is not very high (my original

CD4 count was below 20) but I had it done again in 2011 and it is now 672 which is amazing for someone who is only on herbs.

My weight is now 87kg (180lbs) and I look and feel very healthy and glowing. However the most amazing thing is that my blood test has come back as negative for HIV. It was retested again a second time and was found to still be negative.

God is still a God of miracles!

I continue to work at Eden Herbal Clinic and I am an important part of what we do for the community and the children.

I am part of the girls youth group where I share my testimony with them and teach about different topics like these:

> HIV/AIDS – explanations about the disease.
>
> HIV/AIDS – What is true and what is superstition and rumours.
>
> Say no to sex before marriage.
>
> Helping others with HIV/AIDS
>
> Be a friend to others with HIV/AIDS

I have worked with youth groups through the Catholic Church so I bring this knowledge with me into Eden.

I work with the 0 – 10 year olds, the 11 – 15 year olds and the young adults 16 – 23 year olds.

I have also become a foster mother for a child (Caroline) who was abandoned by her mother at the police station five years ago and I have grown to love her like my own. Caroline is very happy to live with me.

We have now started a support group in the Doma area for the local HIV/AIDS patients and for our workers and children who are positive and I am part of the guidance council for that group. It's about helping others to support themselves and their families and about what happens when the main wage earner or money earner is not there anymore, and how can the woman support her family.

The group started off small but now is up to over 80 people. The different farms have formed smaller support groups and every three months everyone gets together.

We have found that this has really helped people to talk about their disease and to share their knowledge with everyone.

With God's grace I pray that I will still be at Eden in the future, helping people to live positively with HIV/AIDS.

We Treat

But

God

Heals!

REFERENCES AND READING LIST

The following books are the ones we use as references, and are worth having in your library:

Natural Medicine in the Tropics – Anamed
Dr. Hans Martin Hirt, Bindanda M Pia

Margaret Roberts Book of Herbs –
Margaret Roberts

Margaret Roberts - A-Z of herbs
Margaret Roberts

Food Plants of Zimbabwe –
M. H. Tredgold

The Herb Society's Complete Medicinal Herbal
Penelope Ody

The Complete Book of Herbs & Spices.
Lesley Bremness & Jill Norman

Many Thanks

To

Dr. Hans Martin Hirt

Of

ANAMED

Who has analyzed

All the Plants

Used as Medicine

In Africa.

His research has

Advanced Herbal Medicine

Practice and Dosage.

EDEN HERBAL MEDICAL CLINIC HISTORY

Eden Herbal Clinic started because of a medical need in the Doma community. In 2002 the medical care available at the local government facilities was just about nonexistent and there are no private medical facilities closer than three hours away.

An African lady had an abscess on her hand from reaping her corn and her father had approached my husband to ask for assistance with transport to the local hospital which is 25km away. He suggested that maybe she could see me as I am a state registered nurse and that I knew something about herbs. We did manage to treat her hand with herbs and it healed. She was our first patient and so from that day onwards word went around and we started to get people arriving with seriously infected wounds and different diseases, asking for help.

We did not have a facility to cope with the inflow of patients and so we started out on a table under a tree. Eventually in 2004 a group from Goshen Christian Church came out and built a one room building so we could be under some sort of shelter. It was large enough for a wash basin, shelving and four concrete raised beds and a desk. At this stage we will need to add on extra rooms as we have seen 20 000 individual patients to date and our one room is not big enough anymore to try and cope with all the patients.

How the clinic runs today

We have a staff of six people and we run the clinic on a free of charge basis. We open the clinic and treat patients every other day (Monday, Wednesday and Fridays) and the days in between are used for making up the ointments, sourcing, cutting, drying and processing the herbs. Obviously emergencies we don't turn away and cope with them the best way we can. We have to make a judgment and work out if we can deal with the medical situation or transport them to the Mhangura Hospital which is 25km away. However we don't have a special ambulance or vehicle for this so use whatever vehicle may be available.

We keep the costs way down by not using plastic bags to dispense the herbs but use funnels made from scrap paper and use scrap plastic cut into squares for the ointments which are petroleum jelly based. People have to bring their own bottles for liquids like the cough mixtures.

We feel that we would rather the patients use their money to buy nutritious food for their family rather than we take it for a gift that God has given us free of charge in His garden.

Around 80% of our medicine used is herbal. Some of it is bush medicine and some from garden herbs. Unfortunately many people in Zimbabwe today have lost their knowledge of their traditional herbal medicine through westernization and thinking that a tablet or injection is better for you because it's expensive.

It is much easier to just buy a tablet at the pharmacy, than to go out into the bush, pick your leaves and process them to get the result you want. The problem comes when the clinic's, hospitals and pharmacies don't have what you need and so people will get sick or even die from lack of knowledge of what they can use and it's probably right outside their front door.

We also speak to the patients about the spiritual aspect of them wearing strings and beads which they have been given by the local witch doctors for medicine. We will ask them to remove them before we can treat them to break the spiritual bondage they are under. We also council them that Jesus Christ is the person we need to put our faith in and not in a piece of string.

The Clinic works closely with the local clinic and hospital and supplies the hospital with 12lbs of our Herbal Antibiotic Ointment every month. We are registered under the Traditional Medical Practitioners Council of Zimbabwe so that we are legally able to run the clinic and I am still registered as a Registered Nurse.

Herbal medicine is not a new idea. In biblical times there were no pharmacies. Plants are God's medicine chest and an herb is anything that grows. We just don't know what all their benefits are. Aspirin and Digitalis are just two of the drugs derived from plants and we have no idea of how many treatments are still out there.

The plants are also free. You don't have to pay for them. Your child can be treated for a fever by using a wild plant next to your home instead of having to walk 20 miles to get syrup which will cost so much that your family has to go without a meal for a day.

It's lack of **KNOWLEDGE** that is the biggest thief here.

We also run a supplement feeding program to help children in the community with malnutrition. Through this program we also teach nutrition, hygiene and counsel them on what are the right foods and what alternatives they can use for children with malnutrition and what they need to grow. Many of the people are ignorant of that knowledge. They will sell peanut butter or dry beans which are a good protein source for the family and use that money to buy a fizzy drink and white bread which has no real nutritional value and moves them along the road to malnutrition.

The Moringa tree is what is called the miracle tree and is a multi mineral and multi vitamin source. Also a protein source and the seeds can be used for cleaning dirty water. Providing the people with the trees, seeds and educating them on how to use it is essential to show them how herbal medicine can help even in the cases of malnutrition.

We also try and get new born children whose mothers died at birth through the first six months of their lives with formula and then the next six months with high protein foods like peanut butter, beans and eggs. Any child that we have on the supplement feeding program is monitored closely and their weight is taken monthly. We also take the caregivers weight to make sure the food is going where it should be. We have had situations where a nine month old child who weighs only 7 1bs and whom we were supplying the mother with high protein foods and formula, took the items straight from our premises and sell them at the local market.

We try and make the caregiver accountable for the care of the child and we also run a seed program where we give them seeds and cuttings to grow their own health gardens. However we don't have the staff or the time at this stage to follow that project up enough. It's really a whole ministry on its own but it is definitely something we can look at in the future.

We have started a support group for our HIV/AIDS infected workers and their children and our Eden children. This will also grow to include people from the area as there is no other support group operating close by. Mr. Henry Mahogo from the Makondi Christian Hospital will also be involved as he is in charge of the HIV/AIDS outreach program in the area and we work closely with him already.

IMPORTANT DISCLAIMER

Herbs ARE medicine!

Consult your physician before mixing herbal medicines with prescription medications!

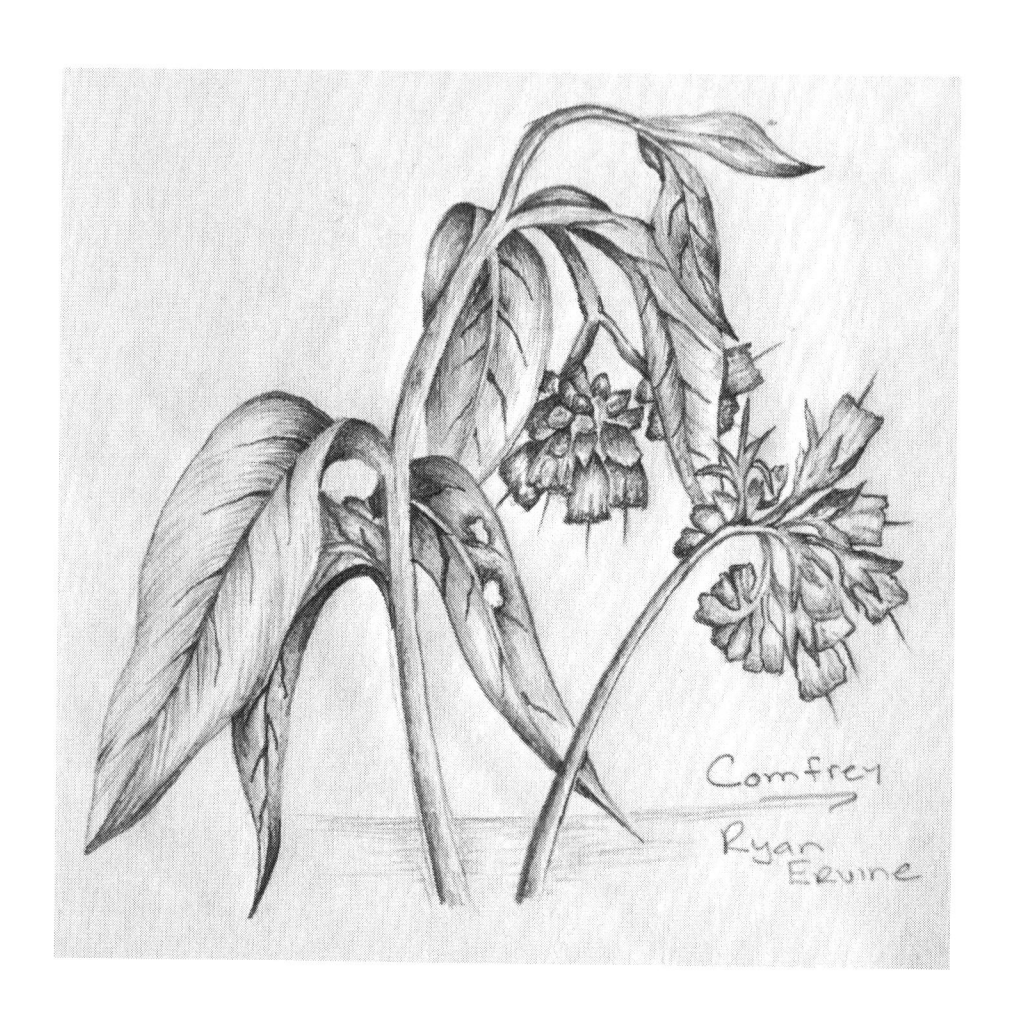

HERBAL REMEDIES & RECIPES

In the pages that follow, we are listing the herbal remedies that we use at the Eden Herbal Medical Clinic.

Abscess

Closed abscess or boil.

- ❖ **Hot compresses** - every two hours over an unopened abscess or boil.

- ❖ **Sugar & Green Soap** – For a closed boil or abscess:-

    Melt one part grated green laundry soap and brown sugar together in a double boiler.
    Mix until the consistency of thick treacle.
    Place this mixture on a cotton pad and when it is the right temp (not too hot but bearable) then place over the area.
    Make sure it is not too hot as you will burn the patient.
    Change this daily.

Open abscess or boil.

- ❖ **Nasturtium leaves** – Clean the area with salt water first then pound the leaves into a paste and bind in place over the affected area that has opened. Put petroleum jelly on the clean skin around the area first as this may burn the normal unaffected area.

- ❖ **Chickweed** – Use this the same way as nasturtiums.

AIDS/HIV

❖ **Ginger and Garlic** – Take half a teaspoon of fresh ginger powder and half a teaspoon of garlic powder together as a tea once a day. It must be as fresh as you can get it.

❖ **Moringa** – One teaspoon of the powder taken three times a day mixed into food or porridge.

❖ **Carrots** – Include plenty of raw carrots in your diet. They contain beta Carotene which is important for your immune system.

❖ **Pumpkin Seeds** – Don't throw away your pumpkin seeds but dry them and add them raw to salads or just eat a handful each week to combat worms and other parasites.

❖ **Garlic** – Use Garlic daily in your diet. Raw is best but much stronger. Garlic is a natural antibiotic and will help your body's defence system to fight disease.

Anaemia

- ❖ **Moringa** – leaf powder is a good source of iron. Use one teaspoon in your porridge or vegetables three times a day.

- ❖ **Iron rich foods** – Eating iron rich foods on a daily basis

    Spinach
    Liver
    Eggs
    Amaranth
    Sweet Potato leaves

- ❖ **Iron pots** – Using iron pots for cooking food especially acid rich foods like tomatoes will draw some of the iron from the pots into the food that is being cooked.

Antibiotic Ointment (Herbal).

This ointment cleans as it heals so is very good for healing wounds after they have been cleaned with the Nasturtium leaves. We have been supplying Mhangura Hospital with a 5litre container every month to use and they use it for everything.

Take 500g Petroleum Jelly (Vaseline)

Add to this container –

Three (3) heaped Tablespoons of finely chopped fresh Basil leaves.

Fifty (50) drops of concentrated Tea Tree Oil.

Mix together and store at room temperature if used quickly or store in a fridge if not used within 3 days.

Anti – Itch Ointment.

(Use for mild skin allergies)

Mix together –

    300g Petroleum Jelly (Vaseline)

    30 drops Eucalyptus oil

    15 drops Lavender Oil

Don't melt the Vaseline before mixing as the oils will evaporate. Mix the oils in the Vaseline tub and store in a cool place.

Use for mild allergy rashes and skin irritations.

Antiseptic Wash

Can be used to clean open wounds, septic sores, and skin grazes.

Mix together –

    4 heaped Tsp of fresh Soapwort

    10 stems of fresh Thyme

    ½ Teaspoon Salt

    1 litre of boiled hot water.

Mix all together in a container and leave to cool down stirring occasionally.

Refrigerate.

Arthritis or Rheumatism

- **Turmeric** – Use turmeric daily in your diet.

- **Cayenne Pepper** – use any of the capsicums in your diet. You can also make a cayenne Pepper ointment which will keep the area warm. Be careful when used on broken skin.

    500g Vaseline
    Three Tablespoon Cayenne pepper powder
    Mix well until smooth.
    Use twice a day on the area.

- **Water** – Drinking plenty of water will help to flush out the joints and help alleviate the build up of uric crystals which cause the pain. At least 2 litres of fresh clean water should be drunk daily.

- **Ginger** – Take up to three teaspoons of ginger in your food daily.

- **Parsley** – This must be included in your daily diet. It is also a diuretic so will help remove the uric acid through your urine.

- **Stinging Nettle** – can be used as an urtication. Use the fresh plant and hit it over the area where the joint is painful. It seems a rather extreme way for treatment but it does alleviate the pain in the joint for a while.

- **Exercise** – Keep exercising. If you stop using the joints it will stiffen up. Use it or lose it as the old saying goes.

- **Vitamins and minerals** – Vitamin C, Vitamin E, and Omega 3 – all are useful for arthritis. Vit C increases the secretion of uric acid. Omega 3 is a joint lubricant and Vitamin E is an antioxidant but don't exceed 400 IU a day.

- **Weight** – Keep your weight down. The heavier you are the more strain your joints take.

- **Diet** – Stay away from sugars, sweet foods, coffee, tea, red meats, bread or yeasty foods, acidic foods like tomatoes, citrus and watch your salt intake. This must become a way of life long wise eating.

Asthma

Don't stop your asthma medications but rather speak to your doctor about using some of these natural treatments along with your medications first.

- **Orange tree leaves** – Boil one tablespoon of chopped cleaned Orange tree leaves in one litre of water for two minutes. Drink 10ml every half an hour through the day to help asthma symptoms.

- **Marjoram** – Take half a teaspoon of dried or freshly chopped leaves, three times a day as a tea infusion. Use honey to taste.

- **Asthma syrup** – see recipe

- **Asthma regime** – see recipe

- **Diet** – Cut out sugars and sweet foods. Be careful of foods with preservatives as this can cause allergies.

- **Water** – drink plenty of fresh water daily. Your body needs to be hydrated.

- **Plantain** – Take half a teaspoon of dried or freshly chopped leaves, three times a day as a tea infusion. Use honey to taste.

- **Stinging Nettle** – Take half a teaspoon of dried or fresh chopped leaves, three times a day as a tea infusion. Use honey to taste.

Asthma Regime

This does not replace asthma medications in serious conditions but does help relieve some of the symptoms and can be used alongside medications.

Mix together: -

    Honey 500ml

    Ginger Mint – chopped – 1 handful

    Sweet Violet leaves – chopped – 1 handful

    Stinging Nettle leaves – chopped – 1 handful

    Aloe Vera sap – (3 leaves) split and the sap scraped off.

    Eucalyptus Leaves – chopped – 1 Tablespoon

Leave to settle for the night. In the morning strain and bottle in glass bottles.

Does not need to be refrigerated if it is to be used within 2 weeks.

Children ages 3 – 5yrs old – 1/2 tsp twice daily

Children ages 6 – 10yrs old – 1tsp twice daily

Adults 1Tbsp twice daily.

Asthma Syrup.

This does not replace asthma medications in serious conditions but does help relieve some of the symptoms and can be used alongside medications.

Boil together:-

    650ml water

    Three large Garlic cloves – chopped finely.

    Boil until the water has boiled away to half the amount.

    Add 120ml Apple Cider Vinegar

    100g of Brown sugar to the above mixture.

    Bottle and refrigerate.

    Children ages 3 – 5yrs old – 1/2 Tsp twice daily

    Children ages 6 – 10yrs old – 1tsp twice daily

    Adults - 1Tbsp twice daily.

Bilharzias

Bilharzias mixture –
Mix together:-

    1 Tablespoon Wormwood
    1 Tablespoon common dock root
    1 Tablespoon Mukwa Bark powder
    1 Tablespoon Parsley

Place contents in a one liter hard plastic container and add 500ml boiling water.

Let soak for half an hour and then add 500ml boiled cool water.

Let soak all night.

Adults – 20ml every hour through the day.

Children – 10 ml every hour through the day.

Continue for the next five days adding more boiled water if needed each night. Then start again with a new herbal mixture.

Continue for two weeks.

Also take one clove of garlic orally three times a day for two weeks. Children take half.

Take orally one tsp Moringa three times a day for two weeks.

Drink plenty of fresh clean water daily.

- **Mukwa bark** *(Pterocarpus Angolensis)* – Used as a tea. Take half a teaspoon three times a day for five days.

- **Wormwood** *(Artemisia annua anamed)* – This herb is a hybrid variety that has been hybridized by the Anamed team.
  Contact them directly through Anamed if you need more information about dosages etc.

  This is one herb we do use in the clinic for Bilharzia and malaria and it works very well.

Breast lumps and pains

This is only temporary treatment. You **MUST** consult your Doctor and he will refer you if need be to see a specialist.

- ❖ **Rue** - Use crushed fresh Rue leaves and rub over the breast area at night. That same night, take 1 tsp crushed fresh Rue leaves and place in 500ml of boiling water. Drink 10 ml. Continue for 3 nights.

- ❖ **Hot compresses** – Use a hot compress over the swelling every 2 hours especially if you are breastfeeding at the time. It could be an abscess forming. Continue to express milk and using a hot compress will help the breast to release milk.

Bronchitis, Flu, Common Cold

Remember flu is a virus and cannot be treated as such. What we are treating are the symptoms or secondary infections from bacteria.

- ❖ **Steam Inhalation** – It's important to use steam inhalation as a way of clearing, draining and opening up the airways. You can use any of the following herbs – Rosemary, Lavender, Mint, Scented geranium, Thyme or to even use all of these together as a scented bowl of steam. Try and do steaming three times a day.

- ❖ **Lemon peel** – Grate a cup of fresh lemon peel and add this to one litre of boiling water.
  Leave to cook for fifteen minutes.
  Strain and drink throughout the day.

- ❖ **Lemon grass** – Boil one cup of fresh or dried chopped lemon grass stalks in 1 litre of water and use the vapour as a steam inhalation. This will help relieve the tightness and wheezing in the chest. Repeat this three times a day.
  You can also drink lemon grass tea using 1 teaspoon of chopped leaves to a mug of boiling water. Take it three times a day and sweeten with honey.

- **Eucalyptus leaves** – Pound 1 handful of the eucalyptus gum tree leaves until mashed and then add this to 1 litre of water which is boiling.
  Drink 1 cup of this mixture three times a day.

- **Ginger** – Take freshly ground ginger as a tea. Use half a teaspoon twice a day as a tea.

- **Garlic** – Take a clove of Garlic three times a day for seven days. This is a natural antibiotic **(remember if you are allergic to sulphur – Garlic has sulphur in it, so use with caution)**

- **Camphor** – Rub Vicks or one of the camphor products on the feet at night and use socks. This will help stop the coughing. Also rub on the chest and back twice a day.

- **Mango or Orange** – Use a tablespoon of the cleaned fresh young leaves chopped and boil them in one litre of boiling water for 10 minutes. Strain and drink 10ml every hour through the day.

- **Tickle cough mixture** – see recipe

- **Garlic & Sugar Mix** (for coughs) – see recipe

- **Cough & Cold Garlic remedy** – see recipe

- **Guava** – Take a tablespoon of new chopped Guava leaves and boil them in one litre of boiling water. Strain and drink through the day <u>OR</u> you can chew a clean new Guava leaf five times a day.

- ❖ **Onions** – Slice Onion rings and put into a dish. Sprinkle brown sugar over them and leave through the night. The juice that comes from this can be used for a cough through the day.

- ❖ **Sweet Wormwood** – Tea made with half a teaspoon of sweet wormwood with a mug of boiling water and sweetened with honey.

- ❖ **Water** – Drink plenty of fluids to keep phlegm loose and easy to cough up. Also to help combat fevers. Use treatments from the coughing, Bronchitis and fever sections.

- ❖ **Rest** – Get plenty of rest and sleep. Your body has to fight this infection and needs rest and sleep to do it.

- ❖ **Diet** – Stay away from sugary foods and foods with lots of preservatives. Don't drink sugared drinks but rather clean fresh water.

Burns

- ❖ **Aloe Vera** – Aloe Vera can be used on recently burned areas. Open up the leaf and place the open end of the area where the gel is against the burnt area. Change this four times a day for the first day then go onto the herbal ointment.

- ❖ **Saline wash** – Two teaspoons of salt in one litre of boiled clean water.
  Use this over the area six times a day to keep it clean.

- ❖ **Herbal Antibiotic Ointment** – see recipe (This must be changed daily)

- ❖ **Paraffin gauze** – Make your own paraffin gauze by layering the open gauze swabs in a clean metal or enamel container.
  Melt the petroleum jelly and when it is melted add a couple of drops of tea tree oil to the liquid.
  Pour this over the gauze and leave it to set.
  Use the paraffin gauze over the ointment before bandaging.

Camphor Rub.

Use this chest rub for flu, colds and bronchitis.

Mix together: -

>500g Petroleum Vaseline.
>Two heaped Tablespoons of finely chopped common garden Mint.
>Fifty drops of camphorated oil or 25 drops of Eucalyptus oil which is stronger.

Mix together and store at room temperature.

Cancer

- ❖ **Garlic** – Eat raw garlic or include garlic in your cooking daily.
  Garlic which is consumed regularly in your diet can help our immune systems combat diseases.

- ❖ **Stress** – Stress is a huge factor in your body's ability to fight disease. A high stress level will affect your immune system's ability to fight disease. You may have to make some tough decisions regarding changing certain areas of your lifestyle.

- ❖ **Cancer syrup** – See recipe

- ❖ **Kigelia** *(Kigelia Africana)* African sausage tree– Take one teaspoon of the dry powder mixed in your porridge or vegetables three times a day.

- ❖ **Diet** – Stay away from sugars, sweet food (e.g. cakes, cookies, candy, sugared pop, sugared gum etc) preservatives (esp. sweeteners)
  Eat plenty of clean organically grown raw foods and salads with natural dressings and olive oil.
  Your body has the ability to fight disease but we destroy its ability to heal itself by the junk we feed it. Junk food has many additives and toxins which limit the bodies ability to heal itself.

- **Hope and positive living** – This is probably more important than the drugs you take. You need to have hope for the future and a positive outlook for the way ahead.

- **Violet** – Chewing violet leaves three times a day is an African remedy for cancer.

Cancer Syrup.

(Use for people with any type of cancer)

Remember this does not rule out normal cancer treatments that your Oncologist suggests but can work alongside the other methods. Check this with your Oncologist.

Mix together –

    500ml Honey or syrup (Honey is better)

    1   large or two small Aloe Vera leaves grated

    1   root of African Potato *(Hypoxis hemerocallidea)* grated

    3 comfrey leaves – chopped

    4 stems of stinging nettle

    4 leaves of sweet violet

    1 Teaspoon Kigelia powder (sausage tree)

    3 Tablespoons either whisky or brandy (alcohol is to make a tincture)

Mix together in a dark plastic or glass container.

Leave for 24 hours. Drain and squeeze out the juice from the herbs into the solution. Place syrup in a sealed dark container in a fridge.

Adults -Take one Tablespoon two times daily.

Candida (thrush)

- **Basil leaves** – As a mouthwash for oral thrush. See the next page for the recipe.

- **Tea Tree Oil – <u>DON'T SWALLOW AS THIS IS TOXIC</u>**
  You can use a couple of drops in warm water as a mouthwash for oral thrush but it must not be swallowed.
  A weak solution can also be used as a douche for vaginal thrush.

- **Thyme** – Thyme tea is really good for people who have a problem with Candida throughout their systems. People who have HIV/AIDS regularly have this problem and this works wonders for their whole body.
  One teaspoon of fresh thyme leaves in a cup of boiling water as a tea and taken three times a day.

Candida (Oral Thrush) Mouthwash

This Basil Mouthwash can be used three times a day.

Mix the following: -

    1 heaped Tsp freshly macerated Basil

    Cup of boiling water.

Or

10 drops of tea tree oil

10ml of warm water.

These can only be used in children old enough to not swallow. For babies and infants it's still best to paint Gentian Violet onto the spots inside the mouth three times a day or you can use one drop of Tea Tree oil on the finger and rub around the inside of a child's mouth.

Cayenne Pepper Ointment.

Can be used for muscular pain, backache, herpes (Shingles - to dry out blisters), sciatica. Be careful when using this on broken skin.

Mix together: -

    500g of Petroleum Vaseline

    3 Tablespoons Cayenne pepper powder.

Mix together until smooth.

This can also be used in combination with the embrocation for muscular pains.

Chicken Pox

- **Chicken pox lotion** – See recipe

- **Neem oil** – Because chicken pox is caused by a virus, Neem oil can help to stop it spreading. Use the oil over the individual spots.

- **Tea tree oil** – Use as a lotion over the individual spots. This can help the itching and also help to dry out the spots.
  Use a few drops in a cup of warm water.

Chicken Pox Lotion

This lotion helps to sooth the itching and also dries out any blisters.

    Mix together: -

        100ml warm water
        10 drops Tea tree oil
        2 drops Eucalyptus oil
        10 drops Lavender Oil

    Mix all together in a container with a lid.

Apply to the spots three times a day but make sure you shake the mixture vigorously before using because the oil will separate from the water.

Conjunctivitis - Sore eyes

- ❖ **Aloe Vera** – Open up a piece of the leaf so that the gel is exposed.
  Place this gel area on the closed eye for five minutes, four times a day.

- ❖ **Camomile** – One handful of flowers added to one litre of boiling water. Filter and use as an eye bath three times a day.

- ❖ **Herbal eye drops** – see recipe

Constipation

- ❖ **Water** – Most people are constipated because they are not drinking enough water. When your body is short of water it will take from your intestines and therefore leaving your stool hard to pass. Drinking a minimum of two litres of water a day will help.

- ❖ **Fennel** – One teaspoon of fennel leaves as a tea three times a day will help. Drink plenty of water as well.

- ❖ **Fresh fruit & Vegetables**– Eating plenty of fresh fruit especially Pawpaw and Mango which have plenty of fibre will also help. Also eat plenty of raw salads and vegetables to help increase the fibre in your diet. Try and stick to cereals with raw oats, bran etc and also use whole grain breads and rolls.

- ❖ **Aloe Vera** – Take a teaspoon of Aloe Vera gel three times a day. It is bitter so mix it with a little honey which will also help constipation.

Adults Cough Mixture

Drinking plenty of water is often the best cure for a cough.

Mix together in an enamel pot over a low heat: -

2 Teaspoons of chopped Eucalyptus leaves

200g Sugar (Brown)

200ml Vinegar (Brown)

2 Tsp Ginger powder

2 Tablespoons Lemon leaves

2 Tablespoons Lemon grass Stir this mixture together.

2 Tsp Garlic.

Stir this mixture together.

Refrigerate

Take 1 tsp three times a day.

Children's Cough Mixture

Drinking plenty of water is often the best cure for a cough.

Mix together: -

Juice of two lemons

200ml honey – (must not be boiled honey and must be pure because of bacteria in the honey comb)

½ Teaspoon Ginger powder

500ml Boiled water

Stir this mixture together.

Refrigerate.

Take 1 tsp three times a day.

If a child is coughing during the night you can give as much as they need.

There is no fear of over dosage as it is a natural remedy.

Cough & Cold Garlic Remedy

Use a strong glass jar and fill with chopped garlic which has been peeled beforehand.
Slowly pour clean Honey into the jar so that it fills the jar properly without leaving gaps between the cloves. Place a lid on the jar but don't screw it down tightly. This will ferment slightly.

Leave in a warm place (i.e. sunny windowsill) for 4 weeks

The honey will absorb the garlic juice and will be ready when you notice the garlic becoming "see through" (opaque) after the four or five weeks is up.

This must be used within 3 months

Dose: Infants: 1/4 (quarter) tsp 2 x Day
       Children 1/2 (half) tsp 2 x Day
       Adult 1 tsp 3 x Day

Garlic & Sugar Mix (For coughs)

Using an enamel pot and mix together: -

300g crushed garlic cloves

500g of brown sugar or honey.

2 lt boiled water.

Wait for 24hrs for the mixture to steep.

Dose: Infants: 1/4 (quarter) tsp 3 x Day

Children 1/2 (half) tsp 3 x Day

Adult 1 tsp 3 x Day

Adults - Lemon & Ginger Cough Mixture

Drinking plenty of water is often the best cure for a cough.

Mix together in an enamel pot: -

> Juice of two lemons
>
> 200ml honey – (must not be boiled honey and must be pure because of bacteria in the honey comb)
>
> ½ teaspoon Ginger powder
>
> 500ml boiled water
>
> 100ml vinegar (brown)
>
> 1 cup Eucalyptus Tea infusion (made beforehand and left to steep until cool).

Stir this mixture together until the sugar has dissolved.

Refrigerate.

Take 1 Tblsp three times a day.

Tickle Cough Mixture

This cough mixture is great for the tickle at the back of the throat. You can use it as much as you need to because it contains natural ingredients.

    1 Part Vinegar (Brown is better)

    1 part Honey (Or use old fashioned brown sugar if no honey)

    1 part water.

    1 part lemon juice

Heat together slowly so the sugar or honey dissolves.

Store in a refrigerator.

Adults – 1 dessert spoon at any time needed.

Children – 1 teaspoon at any time needed.

Diabetes

Don't go off your Diabetic medicines but rather speak to your doctor about using herbs alongside your meds to start with.

- ❖ **Cinnamon** – Cinnamon added to your diet is supposed to regulate your sugar levels. Taking up to two teaspoons a day is the usual amount.

- ❖ **Garlic** – Garlic and onion in your daily diet is a help.

- ❖ **Moringa** – Tea made from the leaves and drunk during the day or by adding the dried Moringa powder to your porridge or cooked vegetables three times a day.

- ❖ **Sore feet** – Use Cayenne pepper ointment but not if the skin is broken because of open sores and wounds. **ONLY USE THIS IF THE SKIN IS NOT BROKEN.** See recipe.

- ❖ **Lemon Grass Tea** – Is supposed to help regulate sugar levels. Take one tsp as a tea three times a day.

Diarrhoea

- **Rehydration Solution** – The biggest danger with diarrhoea is dehydration.

    Mix together: -   1 Litre boiled clean water
    8 teaspoons sugar
    ½ (half) teaspoon salt

    Drink 20 ml every half an hour throughout the day.

- **Rooibos & Mint** – Use one part Rooibos Tea and ½ part mint (fresh or dried). Use one teaspoon of this mixture to one litre of boiling water.

    Drink 20ml every half and hour.

- **Diarrhoea Mixture** – See recipe

- **Diarrhoea Syrup** – See recipe

- **Diarrhoea with blood** – We use our adult diarrhoea mixture but add Mukwa Bark to the mixture.

Diarrhea Mixture.

(Use for mild diarrhea problems)

Mix together: -

    1 Teaspoon Sweet Wormwood

    2 Teaspoons pulverized Mint leaves

    ½ Teaspoon Sunbudzie (*Lannea edulis*) root powder. (Optional)

    ¼ Tsp Salt

    3 Tsp Sugar

OR

    1 Tablespoon Rooibos (*Aspalathus linearis*) Leaf tea

    2 Teaspoons pulverized Mint leaves.

    ¼ Tsp Salt

    3 Tsp Sugar

Add one of the above herbal mixtures to 500ml boiling water in a hard plastic container.

Steep for half an hour and then add 500ml boiled cool water.

Adults - 20ml mixture every half an hour.

Children – 10ml every hour.

Diarrhea Syrup.

(Use for children with mild diarrhea)

Mix together in a dark plastic or glass container: -

    500ml Honey or syrup (Honey is better)

    100g Fresh Wormwood (*Artemisia Absinthian*) pulverized.

Leave for 24 hours.

Drain and squeeze out the juice from the herbs into the solution.

Place syrup in a sealed dark container in a fridge.

Children ages 3 – 5yrs old – 1/4 (quarter) tsp twice daily

Children ages 6 – 10yrs old – ½ (half) tsp twice daily

Adults – 1tsp twice daily.

Diuretic

<u>Don't stop your diuretic medications but rather speak to your doctor about using some of these natural treatments along with your medications first.</u>

- ❖ **Parsley** – Fresh Parsley in your diet especially raw used in salads daily or taken as a tea. Take half a teaspoon three times a day.

- ❖ **Moringa Root Bark** – Take one teaspoon in your porridge or with your vegetables three times a day.

- ❖ **Roselle** (*Hibiscus sabdariffa*) – Tea made from the fruits makes a refreshing tea. You can drink this four times a day.

- ❖ **Rocket** – Rocket taken in salads daily will help as a diuretic.

Ear infections

If there is pus present you must see a doctor.

- ❖ **Herbal ear drops** – See recipes

- ❖ **Garlic** – Take Garlic three times a day as well as using the drops. Garlic is a mild antibiotic.

- ❖ **Shepherds Purse** *-(Capsella bursa-pastoris)* A heaped teaspoon of the chopped herb (seeds, stems and leaves) put into a cup of hot water. Leave to soak and then drink it as a tea through the day and at the same time place a few warm drops of the tea in the ear three times a day with a small piece of cotton wool.

Herbal Ear Drops – Yarrow & Garlic

Can be used for ear pains and minor infections. More serious ear infections with signs of pus must be treated medically.

Mix together : –

    50ml Vinegar.

    50ml Boiled water

    2 Garlic cloves – crushed

    2 Yarrow leaves – chopped fine

Store in a dark bottle and refrigerate

Use as follows: - 0 – 5 yrs 1 drop 3 x daily

                    6 - 12 yrs 2 drops 3 x daily

                    Adults 3 drops 3 x daily

Herbal Ear Drops – Tea Tree

Can be used for ear pains and minor infections. More serious ear infections with signs of pus must be treated medically.

Mix together: –

    10 mls Tea Tree Oil

    50ml Boiled water

    2 Garlic cloves – crushed

    2 Yarrow leaves – chopped fine

Store in a dark bottle and refrigerate

Use as follows: - 0 – 5 yrs 1 drop 3 x daily

                  6 - 12 yrs 2 drops 3 x daily

                  Adults 3 drops 3 x daily

Eczema

- ❖ **Soap** - Stop using normal soap and use the following:-

    Elderberry *(Sambucus nigra)* leaves – One handful of chopped leaves in one litre of boiling water. Let soak for thirty minutes and when the temperature is right use it to wash all over. Let the juice dry on the skin then use the Herbal Antibiotic Ointment as a lotion.
    OR use Aqueous Cream mixed with Tea tree Oil. Do this twice a day.

- ❖ **Aqueous Cream** – Using just a good quality Aqueous Cream instead of soap for washing is enough to lessen the Eczema.

- ❖ **Cabbage** – Liquidised Cabbage leaves and used as a lotion can bring relief to the itchiness.

- ❖ **Aloe Vera** – Open up the leaf and wipe the juice and gel over the affected area. It will stop the itchiness and has a cooling effect on your skin.

- ❖ **Bulbinella** *(Bulbine frutescens)* **Juice** – Can be used the same as Aloe Vera.

- ❖ **Sodium Bicarb** – You can put it in the bath water or make a paste with a little water to put over the affected areas.

- ❖ **Soapwort (Bouncing Bess)** – Crush the leaves and rub with a little water to make a soapy liquid and rub over the affected area. Leave it to dry on the area and this will help take away some of the itchiness.

- ❖ **Rooibos Tea** – Taken internally as a tea and also using the tea as a wash and leaving it to dry on the skin will help.

- ❖ **Diet** – Cut out sugars, high citrus and acid intake (e.g. Strawberries, Oranges, Tomatoes) Dairy products and wheat, eggs, and food additives can also be known to worsen the condition.

- ❖ **Chickweed** – Chop the leaves and use a cup of leaves to 500ml of boiling water. Use this as a wash twice a day. Leave the juice to dry on the skin before using the lotion of your choice.

Embrocation.

This herbal oil can be used for muscular pain, sciatica, menstrual cramping, stomach pains, scarring from Herpes etc

Collect together : -

> 1 part Rosemary (Can use leaves and flowers)
> 1 part Lavender (can use leaves and flowers)
> 1 part Scented Geranium *(Pelargonium graveolens)* leaves.

Chop as small as possible and mix together.

Then mix with: -

1 teaspoon ginger powder
1 teaspoon of Black Pepper.

Place in a large glass jar with a tight lid and pack the herbs into the jar without packing them down too hard (you need to leave some air space between for the oil to enter) Fill up the jar with either sunflower oil or a vegetable oil. Don't fill the jar to the top with the oil as you need to leave space for fermentation. Leave a gap of around 1 ½ Inches.
Add 6 drops of pure eucalyptus oil to the jar.
Close down your jar tightly and place on a sunny windowsill for around 30 days **OR** you can place the jar in a warming draw at a very low heat for 5 days. Make sure the lid is not plastic if the warming draw is very hot. Strain and bottle the oil.

Epilepsy treatment

This must not be used instead of medications but only if the person cannot afford the tablets or cannot get to them

There are also a few traditional plants locally that are used to treat epilepsy, and we are looking into those at the moment.

Mix together: -

    1 level teaspoon of chopped fresh Rue Leaves

    500ml boiling water

Mix all together in a container.

Take 1 teaspoon of the mixture three times a day.

Beware:- Rue can cause LIVER & KIDNEY DAMAGE if used the wrong way.

Eye Drops

Can be used for sore eyes, irritated eyes, tired eyes and not serious eye infections. **Any sign of pus in the eye or injury must be treated medically by a professional.**

Mix together: –

    200ml **Boiled** clean water

    Pinch of salt

    1 Teaspoon chopped cleaned herbs – (either Chick weed, Black jack or Borage)

Use as follows: - 0 – 5 yrs 1 drop 3 x daily

                      6 - 12 yrs 2 drops 3 x daily

                      Adults 3 drops 3 x daily

This mixture must be made daily and not kept over from one day to the next. It does sting when first administered but is very good for allergies esp. the chick weed solution.

Be **VERY** careful where you collect your plants and that the area is not polluted by passing vehicles or by animal manure.

Fever

- **Yarrow** – Use the chopped fresh or dried leaves as a tea and take three times a day. See notes on Yarrow.

- **Lippia Tea** *(Lippia javancia)* – This is a wild plant. Use the powder the same as above.

- **Makoni Tea** *(Fadogia ancylantha)* – This is a wild plant. Use the powder the same as above.

- **Wild Willow** *(Salix mucronata)* – Use the powder of the willow leaves or bark. Take only half a teaspoon three times a day but be careful and only use it for people over the age of sixteen years as it has properties like Aspirin and should be taken with food to prevent gastric problems.

- **Lemon Grass** – A teaspoon of either chopped fresh lemon grass or the dried powder taken with a cup of boiling water three times a day. This is very refreshing.

- **Water** – Drinking plenty of fresh plain water will also help a fever. Up to four litres through the day because you will be sweating as well.
  Children 1 - 2 litres.

- **Sow Thistle** *(Sonchus olearceus)* – Use for fevers. The whole plant can be taken raw or in salads.

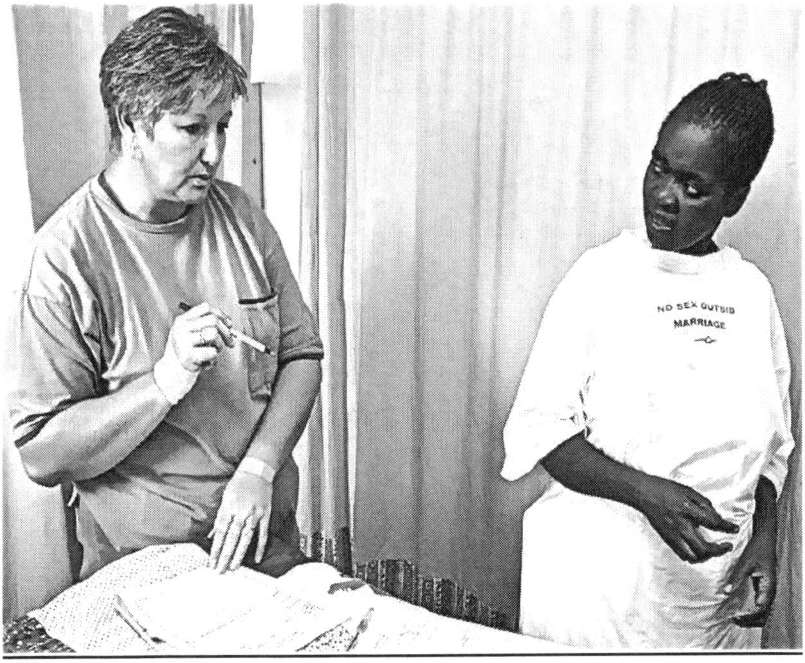
NO SEX OUTSID
MARRIAGE

Fungal Infections

One of the secrets of curing Fungal Infections is not to stop the treatment too early. If possible continue the treatment for at least another week after its looking better.

- ❖ **Garlic** – Crush fresh garlic and place it over the area with a plaster. Change this daily but be very careful as fresh garlic can burn the skin. Don't layer it on too thick and watch for redness. You will need to stop if it is irritating the skin. Also you can only use this for small ringworm of other fungal areas.

- ❖ **Pawpaw** – The white latex from the unripe fruit of the Paw Paw fruit mixed with a little vegetable oil will also work for fungal infected areas. Use about twenty drops of the latex with 100ml of sunflower oil.

- ❖ **Onion** – A peeled onion layer placed over the area and bound in place. Change daily.

- ❖ **Tea Tree Oil** – Use pure Tea Tree Oil and rub a drop into the area every couple of hours. For children you must dilute it a little with sunflower oil.

Gastritis

- ❖ **Aloe Vera** – Boiling a cup of finely chopped leaves in a litre of boiling water. Drink this mixture twice a day. Use honey to taste if you need to as the Aloe juice can be very bitter.

- ❖ **Ginger** – Use fresh grated ginger or fresh ginger powder. Take half a teaspoon in a cup of boiling water as a tea three times a day. Use honey to taste.

- ❖ **Mint** – Mint tea will help with gastric pains. Take half a teaspoon of chopped mint leaves in a cup of boiling water. Sip this slowly over a twenty minute period.

- ❖ **Dill** – Taken as a tea as above or included in your daily diet.

- ❖ **Bicarb of Soda** – Take a teaspoon in a glass of water three times a day will work to neutralise the acid in the stomach and lessen the pain.

- ❖ **Black Jack** - Use one teaspoon of the chopped plant to a cup of boiling water as a tea. Use honey to taste. You can have this three times a day.

Haemorrhoids

Haemorrhoids affect a lot more people than we realise. They are actually varicose veins in the anus and can be internal or external. It's the external ones that are so uncomfortable.

A difficult childbirth can also cause Haemorrhoids.

- **Yarrow** – See recipe for Yarrow Ointment.

- **Water** – having a warm sitz bath and being able to soak that area will bring relief. Adding Tea Tree oil or a strong lemon grass tea to the water may also bring relief. Also make sure you drink plenty of fresh water to prevent constipation.

- **Worms** – Haemorrhoids can be a sign of internal worm infestation so do the treatment for worms first.

- **Diet** – Make sure you are eating plenty of fibre, fresh fruits and vegetables to prevent constipation.

- **Aloe Vera** – The gel placed on some cotton wool and put over the area will cool and soothe the itchiness. Change every hour.

- **Witch Hazel** – Soak a cotton pad with Witch Hazel and place over the haemorrhoids. Change hourly. This will soothe and cool the area and help with the itchiness.

- ❖ **Chickweed** – Macerate the stems and leaves until like a paste. Use this as a dressing on the haemorrhoids with a pad. This will relieve the irritation. Change twice a day.

- ❖ **Capsicums** – Add capsicums (Cayenne Pepper, Chilli etc) to your diet. There are certain fungi in your bowel that can cause haemorrhoids and the Capsicums will help control it.

- ❖ **Elands Bean (***Elephantorrhiza Elephantina***)** – This is a wild plant and the root is used. Place a small piece of the fresh root between your back bottom molar and gum and leave it here for 12 hours. Suck continuously on it throughout the day.

Hemorrhoid - Soothing Bath Oil

To relieve hemorrhoid pain: -

You will need to have available:-

> 6 drops Eucalyptus oil
>
> 6 drops Chamomile oil
>
> 3 drops Mint oil
>
> 20 drops good vegetable oil

Add a teaspoon of this mixture to warm water in a hip bath and use this as a sitz bath.

Bathe for 5 – 10 minutes.

After bathing use some of the oil and dab over the affected area with a piece of cotton wool.

Headache

- ❖ **Water** – Most headaches are caused by a too low intake of water. Our bodies need a minimum of two litres of clean water every day. This does not include tea, coffee, alcohol etc.

- ❖ **Rosemary** – One teaspoon of chopped fresh or dried leaves in a cup of boiling water as a tea. Use honey to taste. You can take this three times a day.

- ❖ **Stress** – Don't ever underestimate the effect that stress has on your body. This can also be the cause of headaches. Take time to smell the roses or at least take time out to sit and breathe in the aroma of your herbal tea.

- ❖ **Lemon Grass** – One teaspoon of chopped fresh or dried leaves in a cup of boiling water as a tea. Use honey to taste. You can take this three times a day.

- ❖ **Willow** – Take half teaspoon twice a day with food. This is a type of Aspirin so also taking quarter Aspirin twice a day with food over a ten day period along with plenty of food can help. This has also been known to help migraines.

Heart Disease (Hypertension etc)

Don't stop your heart medications but rather speak to your doctor about using some of these natural treatments along with your medications first.

- ❖ **Garlic** – Included in your diet on a daily basis is supposed to lower blood pressure and help fight cholesterol. This includes onions as they come from the same family.

- ❖ **Stress** – Don't underestimate the effect stress can have on your body. If you are under a great deal of stress and have heart problems you will need to seek help through a counsellor or a doctor.

- ❖ **Calcium** – A lack of calcium in the body can cause high blood pressure. Taking calcium along with garlic over a period of fourteen days will show you whether this is the problem. Take one clove of garlic and one tablet of calcium (600mg) twice a day with food.

- ❖ **Willow** – Using a low dose of willow twice a day will also help prevent some serious heart problems. Use half a teaspoon twice a day with food. (We have found that many local people cannot afford the blood pressure tablets so we needed to come up with something to aid prevention)

- ❖ **Parsley** – As a diuretic. Take half a teaspoon of fresh parsley as a tea three times a day but also include fresh parsley in your daily diet.

- **Rosemary** – Can lower blood pressure in hypertensive patients but can also raise blood pressure in hypotensive patients. Take it as a tea using half a teaspoon in a cup of boiling water. Take this three times a day.

- **Lions Ears** *(Leonotis leonurus)* – A wild plant which grows in the rainy season. Make a tea infusion from the leaves and roots and take this 3 x day.

Heart Problems – Care for the heart

* **Baths** - Warm relaxing baths with lemon Balm leaves added to the water help to soothe.

* **Exercise** - Exercise for 20 minutes a day in the fresh air to oxygenate the blood and strengthen the heart.

* **Caffeine** - Avoid coffee if you have cardiac problems. The caffeine it contains will cause tachycardia (rapid heart-beat).

***Smoking** - Give up smoking; it harms both the heart and circulatory system.

* **Lemon**- Drink a glass of water containing two tablespoons of sugar and a dash of lemon juice to ease cardiac palpitations.

***Cayenne pepper** - has also been known to help regulate heart beat. Take ¼ tsp and chase it down with water.

Heart Stress Reducing Lemon Balm Tea

This tea will help to soothe and calm the heart when under stress.

Mix together in a bowl: -

> 20g dried Lemon balm leaves
>
> 20g dried Rue leaves
>
> 20g Caraway seeds
>
> 20g dried Lavender leaves
>
> 20g dried Rosemary Leaves

Mix the herbs and store in an air tight container.

To make the tea, add one heaped teaspoon of the mixture to 200ml hot water and leave to infuse for 20 minutes.

Strain and add honey to sweeten, if desired.

Drink up to 2 cups daily.

This is a very relaxing tea and will help soothe stress as well.

Herbal Oils

- ❖ **Basic herbal oils** – Using macerated herbs in a glass bottle with good quality sweet oil or almond oil is how you make basic herbal oil.
  Because the sweet oils are too expensive locally a sunflower cooking oil can be used instead.

  Use 1 part herbs to 1 part oil. The herbs must be chopped or macerated. Don't fill the glass bottle to the top as the mixture will ferment slightly. Leave in a warm place like on a sunny windowsill for up to two weeks.
  Strain, bottle and keep in a dark place.
  Preferably use glass bottles to store the oil so it is not contaminated.

  Herbs that you can use:

  Lavender
  Rosemary
  Scented geranium
  Lemon Grass
  Lemon Verbena
  Sweet Violet Flowers
  Lemon Peel
  Crushed Vanilla Pods
  Rose petals from scented roses
  Jasmine flowers
  Honey suckle flowers

  Any leaves or flowers with a perfume

You can also mix together which ones you want to make your own scented oil.

Use as a massage oil or a bath oil.

A quicker way you could also heat gently in a double boiler. Stirring regularly. Leave to simmer for up to half an hour (must not over boil). Strain through muslin or a thin cotton cloth. Bottle the oil in glass bottles and keep in a dark cupboard.

- ❖ **Rosemary** – This oil has always been used for hair conditioning. Massage the rosemary oil into your hair once a week and leave it for half an hour before washing with shampoo.

- ❖ **Muscle oil** – See our Embrocation recipe

- ❖ **Clove Oil** – Make with freshly crushed cloves and olive oil. 1 part of each.
  Leave in a warm place for up to a month.
  You can use this for toothache

Herbal vinegars

- ❖ **Basic herbal Vinegar** – Use any kind of vinegar but the better quality vinegar you use then better the end product. Choose which herb or herbs you want to flavour it with. Use only fresh herbs for the vinegar. You can use any of the following:-

    Marjoram
    Oregano
    Basil
    Bay Leaves
    Chillies
    Celery
    Dill
    Fennel
    Garlic
    Mint Varieties
    Parsley
    Rosemary
    Thyme

    You can combine the ones you want to use to flavour the vinegar. Change the fresh leaves every three weeks. Leave the vinegar on a sunny windowsill until it reaches the flavour you need. You may need to experiment with what goes together best and how useful it will be for cooking.

Herpes

- **Cayenne** – See recipe for Cayenne Ointment. This ointment helps to dry out the blisters and will heal them quickly.

- **Embrocation** – See recipe for embrocation. Because the Herpes virus affects the nerves the pain can go on for up to two years. The embrocation massaged into the area three times a day will help alleviate some of that pain.

- **Lemon Juice** – fresh lemon Juice squeezed onto a cold sore several times a day will help dry out the lesion quickly.

Insect Bites & Stings

- ❖ **Ice** – The first treatment for any sting or bite. You need to keep the ice on the area for at least fifteen minutes. The problem is there may not always be ice available where you are at the time.

- ❖ **Comfrey** – Fresh Comfrey leaves macerated and rubbed on the area will help relieve the pain.

- ❖ **Mint** – Rubbing macerated mint onto insect bites or stings will help take the pain away.

- ❖ **Borage** – Crushed leaves rubbed onto insect bites and stings will help with the pain and any allergies.

- ❖ **Sodium Bicarbonate** – made into a paste with water and placed over the sting or bite will relieve some of the pain.

- ❖ **Bulbinella** – Squeeze the juice from the leaves onto the area. It will bring instant relief.

- ❖ **Aloe Vera** – use the juice over the area. This will help soothe the pain and the itch.

Insect Repellents

- **Herbs** – Use stalks of dried basil, lavender, lemon grass on open fires while outside in the evening to deter mosquitoes and other insects.

- **Citronella Oil** – Has always been one of the deterring oils for mosquitoes. You will need to dilute it with olive oil for a body rub or you can burn the oil as a lamp close to where you are sitting.

- **Basil** – Hanging bunches of basil around the kitchen will deter flies or having a plant of Basil in a pot on a sunny windowsill will work the same way. You will need to bruise a few leaves every day to release the odour.

- **Khakibos** *(Targets minuata)* – Use it the same way as basil. You can also put fresh Khakibos in the dog's beds to deter fleas. Rubbing chopped up Khakibos onto their coats will also deter fleas and ticks.

- **Tansy** – Hanging bunches of Tansy in the kitchen will keep the flies away. You can also use it the same way as Khakibos for the dogs.

- **Spray** – Mix together one cupful of chopped up African marigold, Khakibos and Tansy and add to 5 litres of boiling water. Leave to soak overnight and strain. Use this for spraying fruit trees, pumpkins and cucumbers for stinging insects.

- ❖ **Rue** – Use this the same way as you would use Khakibos.

- ❖ **Wormwood** – Is repellent to moths so can be dried and made into sachets for linen closets.

- ❖ **Peppermint** – Rubbing crushed peppermint leaves onto your skin will repel mosquitoes. Test it first as your skin may be sensitive to the oils in the herb. Hanging Peppermint branches in the kitchen will also keep the flies away.

Insomnia

- **Hot bath** – Taking a hot bath before retiring in the evening and using one of the herbal bath oils will help you sleep.

- **Lavender** – Taken as a tea half an hour before going to bed will help to relax you after a busy day. Take a teaspoon of lavender in a mug of boiling water. Also making yourself a lavender flower and leaf pillow which you can sleep on at night will help.

- **Caffeine** – Stay away from caffeine drinks from midday onwards.

- **Scented geranium** – Use the scented leaves to make a pillow to sleep on.

Jaundice

This does not take the place of initial treatments for hepatitis or other liver problems. Rather it's to help you recover afterwards. Please check with your doctor.

- ❖ **Pawpaw (Papaya)** – Eating unripe Pawpaw fruit will help the symptoms of liver problems. Cook and eat it as a vegetable. This is a liver cleanser and will help get rid of toxins. At the same time stay away from fatty foods and drink plenty of water and glucose water.

- ❖ **Glucose** – Glucose solution made up with ten teaspoons of sugar in two litres of water. Drink through the day. Repeat daily for seven days.

- ❖ **Parsley** – Having fresh Parsley in your diet will also help recovery from liver disease. At least quarter a cup of fresh parsley should be eaten daily and a strong tea taken once a day.

- ❖ **Elderberry** – Make a tea using elder flowers. A quarter cup of elder flowers and filled with boiling water. Taken twice a day and sweetened with honey.

- ❖ **Rosemary** – Taken as a tea using half a teaspoon in a cup of boiling water. Take this three times a day.

Kidney disease & UTI

- **UTI(Urinary Tract Infections)regime**– See recipe

- **Parsley** – Parsley is a slight diuretic and so is beneficial when you have water retention. Include it in your diet and also take it as a tea. Half a teaspoon in a cup of boiling water. Take this three times a day for a week then take a break for three days and continue. Don't go longer than a week at a time.

- **Water** – Drinking plenty of water and staying away from sugar and sugared juices and foods can also help.

- **Cranberry Juice** – Cranberry juice is high in Vitamin C and along with plenty of clean water can flush out the infection.

- **Prevention** – If you are susceptible to bladder infections you need to look at prevention.
  Cut back or even out of sugar and sugared drinks and foods.
  Also be careful of too much bread made from yeast. Too much seems to lower resistance to yeast infections.
  Don't use G String underpants or thongs as this has a wick effect for bacteria from the anal area to the urinary area.
  Other preventative measures are listed under the UTI regime recipe.

- ❖ **Celery** – Celery leaves are slightly diuretic.
    Make a tea using half a teaspoon of chopped leaves to a cup of boiling water.
    Take twice a day for seven days, take a break and then resume as needed.
    Don't go for longer than a week at a time.

Lactation

- **Water** – Locally we have found that new mothers who don't have much milk may not be drinking enough water. Increased water consumption usually increases the milk.

- **Fennel** – Fennel tea taken three times a day. Take a teaspoon in a cup of boiling water. This will increase the breast milk.

- **Diet** – We have found one of the main problems is in the diet. The mother is not getting the right foods or not enough food. Increase proteins, fresh fruits and vegetables and the quality of her breast milk will increase.

Weaning

- **Parsley** – Put fresh parsley in the bra cup against the nipple will dry out the breasts when you need to start weaning your child.
  Change this twice a day. We use this at the clinic and it does work.

Malaria

- **Wormwood** *(Artemisia annua anamed)* – This herb is a hybrid variety that has been hybridized by the Anamed team.
  Contact them directly through Anamed if you need more information about dosages etc.

  This is one herb we do use in the clinic for Bilharzia and malaria and it works very well.

Menstruation Problems

- ❖ **Parsley & Yarrow** – For excessive bleeding, use one part of each.
  Mix together and use one teaspoon of the mixture as a tea three times a day.

- ❖ **Willow** – Take willow twice a day. Half a teaspoon twice a day with food. This is for dysmenorrhoea (period Pains)

- ❖ **Hot Compresses** – Using a hot water bottle over the lower abdomen will be soothing for period pains. Curling up in a foetal position on your side with the hot water bottle will also help.

- ❖ **Embrocation** – Massaging the embrocation over the lower abdomen after doing the hot water bottle will help. See the recipe for embrocation.

Migraine

- **Feverfew** – This is an age old remedy for migraine sufferers but needs to be taken daily and not just when the migraine is coming on.
  Eat 3 small leaves daily over a year.

- **Willow** (Aspirin) - Over a long term period. Taking a quarter tablet or half a teaspoon of willow on a daily basis can help migraine sufferers.
  Don't forget to take it with food.

Nausea

- **Ginger** – This is probably the best known herb for nausea. Fresh is best and half a teaspoon of grated ginger in a mug of boiling water and sipped slowly will help. If no fresh ginger then use powdered Ginger as fresh as you can find.

- **Lemon Grass** – A cup of lemon Grass tea will also help with nausea. Use a teaspoon of chopped leaves to a mug of boiling water as a tea. Sip it slowly.

- **Mint** – A cup of mint tea will help nausea as well. Take it the same way as above.

- **Basil** – A weak solution of basil leaves taken as a tea will help nausea. Use half a teaspoon or even a quarter to a mug of boiling water. Use honey to taste.

Oedema

<u>**Don't stop your diuretics if you have a serious medical condition but rather speak to your doctor about using some of these natural treatments along with your medications first.**</u>

- **Parsley** – Include fresh parsley in your diet especially in fresh salads every day. You can also take a tea using a teaspoon of freshly chopped parsley in a cup of boiling water as a tea and taken three times a day. Take for 1 week then have a break of three days and repeat. Don't take it for longer than 7 days at a time without a break.

- **Carrots** – The tops of the carrots can be used to replace parsley in salads or added. They belong to the same family.

- **Rocket** – Is also a diuretic and taken fresh in salads on a daily basis will help oedema.

- **Maize hair** – (corn hair) Take a teaspoon of chopped maize hair in a cup of boiling water as a tea. Use honey to taste.
  Take this three times a day.

- **Dandelion Root** – Take a teaspoon of Dandelion Root in a cup of boiling water as a tea.
  Take this three times a day.

Poisoning

<u>If the patient is unconscious get emergency help as soon as you can. This is serious. But if the patient is conscious and you are far from help there are a few things you can do.</u>

- **Charcoal Powder** – If you have an idea that the person has drunk poison or has swallowed anything that could poison him like plants etc use charcoal powder mixed with milk. A teaspoon of charcoal powder to half a cup of milk. Repeat every half an hour. The charcoal will bind to the poison and neutralize it as it works its way through the system. Monitor them closely and treat symptomatically. You can use charcoal from wood fires. Grind it into a powder.

- **Castor Oil** *(Ricinus communis)* – <u>**NEVER make a person vomit who has swallowed Paraffin, Diesel or petrol.**</u>
  If they inhale these products they will do more damage. Give castor oil for people who have eaten plants that are toxic.
  Adults - 2 tsp twice a day
  Children - 1 tsp twice a day and get help as soon as you can.
  Babies – get them to a medical person urgently

Scabies

- ❖ **Hygiene** – Prevention is always better than cure and the reason why most people get scabies is through bad hygiene. Washing blankets once a week and putting them out in the sun during the day will help. Putting the mattress or sleeping mat in the sun during the day also helps. Daily baths with soap or using soapwort and clean clothes will also prevent scabies infestation. Unfortunately when one person has it most will get it in the family.

- ❖ **Oil for scabies** – Mix one part Paraffin and one part vegetable oil. The patient must bath twice a day and rub the oil into the skin when they are dry. Continue this for three days.

- ❖ **Sickle Bush** (*Dichrostachys cinerea*) – This is a wild tree. Make an ointment from the seed pod and use it twice a day for 5 days.

Sexually Transmitted Diseases

(Mainly Pelvic Inflammatory Diseases, Thrush)

Mix together in an enamel container: -

    1 Large tbsp chopped parsley leaves.

    ½ tbsp Rooibos leaves

    3 cloves Garlic – crushed

    3 large Nasturtium leaves – chopped.

Add to this 500ml boiling water and let steep for half an hour, then add 500ml boiled cool water.

Drink 20ml of this mixture every hour. At night add another litre of boiling water to the mixture and steep overnight again.

Drink the same quantity the next day – continue for 5 days and then start the process all over again with a fresh batch of herbs and continue for 2 weeks.

Take 1 clove of Garlic orally three times a day with food for 2 weeks.

Take 1 Tsp Moringa Powder with food orally three times a day for 2 weeks.

For the woman use a garlic pessary every two days for 2 weeks (Peel the clove before insertion) a condom must be used during treatment and the partner must also be treated. They must wash twice daily

If genital sores are also present then use the Herbal Antibiotic Ointment three times a day and sit in a sitz saline bath two times a day.

Strokes

Don't stop your medications but rather speak to your doctor about using some of these natural treatments along with your medications first.

- ❖ **Care and love** – This is the best medicine for anyone. To know that they are loved and cared for no matter what their medical condition is.
  Having a stroke can be a very frightening experience because the patient feels they are not in control anymore.

- ❖ **Prevention** – prevention is always better than a cure but sometimes people don't know that they have medical conditions that may cause a stroke (e.g. Hypertension). In the rural areas in Doma most people have never had their blood pressure taken or even seen a doctor. High blood pressure must be treated and the patients can be given low doses of willow to take over a long period.

- ❖ **Diet** – Lose weight if you are overweight and cut back on sugars, fats, salt and alcohol. Make sure you eat plenty of fresh salads, fruit and vegetables on a daily basis.

- ❖ **Garlic** – Use Garlic daily in the diet as it can lower blood pressure.

- ❖ **Rosemary** – Rosemary tea has been known to lower blood pressure. Take a teaspoon of leaves in a cup of boiling water. Take this three times a day.

- **Capsicums** – Included in your diet will help strengthen blood vessels.

Toothache

These are only temporary measures as you will need to see a dentist at some stage and either have the tooth treated or pulled. Most people out where we are have them pulled as they don't have the money for treatments.

Obviously an abscess will need antibiotics but you can also include these treatments along with the antibiotic.

- ❖ **Salt** – A hot salt mouthwash taken every two hours. As hot as you can bear it in your mouth and held against the painful tooth.
  1 teaspoon of salt to a cup of hot water.

- ❖ **Clove** – Clove oil dropped on the tooth will help the pain. Do this three times a day.

- ❖ **Yarrow** – Use a piece of leaf and pack it into the hole in the tooth. Change twice a day.

- ❖ **Sweet Wormwood** – Use a piece of leaf and pack it into the hole in the tooth. Change twice a day.

- ❖ **Lemon Grass** – Chewing a fresh leaf every two hours with the affected tooth will ease some of the pain.

- ❖ **Rue** – Use a piece of leaf and pack it into the hole in the tooth. Change twice a day.

- ❖ **Thorn Apple** *(Datura stramonium)* – This is a wild plant and is **toxic** so care must be taken. The juice from the green seed pod is used.
  1 drop is dropped into the hole in the tooth. Apparently it kills the nerve in the tooth and so gets rid of the pain.
  Angela has used this treatment herself when she was in agony from toothache and it worked.

- ❖ **Herbal Toothpaste** – See recipe

Toothpaste (herbal)

Staying away from sugar, sugary foods and refined foods is the best preventative toothpaste.

Mix together: -

    1 part finely ground Eucalyptus Powder

    1 part fine salt or Bicarb of Soda.

Mix together and seal the container well so that the contents stay dry.

Can be used to replace ordinary toothpaste.

Tuberculosis

Don't stop your medications but rather speak to your doctor about using some of these natural treatments along with your medications first.

- **Mukwa** *(Pterocarpus Angolensis)* – Burn the root bark and use the ash.

    Take 1 teaspoon of this ash three times a day.
    Also use the Mukwa bark powder and drink ½ tsp of the powder as a tea three times a day.

- **Garlic** – One clove taken three times a day for two weeks at a time will help with the coughing.

- **Hibiscus (rosella)** – Taking a tea from the flower capsules three times a day. This is high in Vitamin C and will help build immune systems. Usually one of the first signs for a person having HIV/AIDS is Tuberculosis.

UTI regime

Mix together: -

    2 large tablespoons chopped parsley

    ½ tablespoon Rooibos leaf tea

    3 nasturtium leaves – chopped

    ½ tsp ginger powder

    3 pieces rosemary

    1 teaspoon Moringa leaves chopped or powder

Place contents in a 1 lt hard plastic container and add 500ml boiling water.

Let steep for half an hour and then add 500ml boiled cool water.

Drink 20ml of this mixture every half an hour.

At night add another 1 lt of boiling water to the herbs and let steep all night. Continue for the next five days and then start again with a new herbal mixture.

Continue for 2 weeks.

At the same time take the following: -

Take 1 clove of garlic orally three times a day for 2 weeks

Take orally 1 Tsp Moringa three times a day for 2 weeks.

Drink plenty of fresh clean water daily. At least 2 lt minimum a day.

Always remember hygiene. Esp. woman

* Always urinate and wash after intercourse.

* After being on toilet always wipe from front to back.

* Try and wash after bowel movements esp. if you are susceptible to urinary tract infections.

* Don't wear G string under wear. They act as a "wick" for bacteria to move from the anal area to the urinary tract.

* Always drink plenty of fresh water daily. At least 2lt minimum.

Venereal Diseases.

❖ **Prevention** – This really is a case for prevention is better than cure and this is where morals come into discussion.
 One partner for life and wait till marriage before having sexual intimacy, but the modern thinking is much more loosely veiled and it's a case of "if it feels good then do it" However there is a price to pay and many people become sterile from picking up venereal Diseases when younger.
Let's teach our children God's way first before the world teaches them its way.

❖ **STD Regime** – See recipe

❖ **Genital Sores** – Take a sitz bath twice a day and use the herbal Antibiotic Ointment. Also put them onto the STD regime – See recipe. Both partners must be treated.

❖ **Aloe Vera** – Cut the leaf to get the gel and rub the gel into the sores every two hours.

❖ **Horn Pod Tree** *(Diplorhynchus condylocarpon)* – This is a medium sized wild tree. The roots are dried and made into a powder. Half a teaspoon is taken orally 3 x day.

Vomiting

- **Rooibos & Mint** – use a teaspoon of Rooibos tea with a teaspoon of chopped mint in a cup of boiling water.
  Drink 20 ml of this mixture every half an hour.
  Children can drink 10ml every half an hour.
  Keep the amounts small but often.

- **Ginger** – Use fresh grated ginger or freshly ground ginger.
  Use half a teaspoon in a cup of boiling water as a tea.

Warts & Verruca's

- **Wart Ointment** – See recipe (this treatment can take quite a while to work but it can also act quickly depending on the wart.
  We even used it on my sister's dog's nose that had a wart on it and it worked a treat.

- **Garlic** – Crushed garlic placed over the wart with a cotton pad and bound in place will burn the wart and get rid of it. However some people's skin may be sensitive to the garlic and it will blister so be careful. Change daily until the wart drops off.

- **Verruca's** – These are actually warts which are growing inwards. Use a blade (scalpel blade or a clean razor blade) and scrape them twice a day. They will disappear.

- **Asthma weed** *(Euphorbia hirta)* – This plant grows wild in gardens and can become a pest in some areas. It exudes a white latex when the stem is broken. Dabbing that latex on the warts three times a day will get rid of them.

- **Dandelion** – The juice from the stem can be rubbed on the wart 3 x day.

Wart Ointment

Can be used on Genital warts as well as ordinary warts on hands and feet.

Mix together: -

>   300g Petroleum Jelly.

>   80 drops Tea Tree Oil

>   5 heaped teaspoons of crushed aspirin (325mg)

Mix all together well and store in a container at room temperature.

For genital warts it's always better for the patient to have a sitz bath first in warm salty water and then to dry the area and apply the ointment twice times a day.

They must always use a clean cloth for drying and no one else must use this cloth otherwise they could be infected.

Worms

- **Garlic** – Take a spoonful of chopped garlic each morning for five days on an empty stomach.

- **Pumpkin Seeds** – dried pumpkin pips taken each week will help prevent a build up of parasites in the system. For tape worm take a handful of seeds, chew thoroughly and follow this with castor oil (2 tablespoons) after half an hour. The pumpkin seeds apparently paralyse the tape worm so it loses its hold and the castor oil gets it out of the system.

- **Herbal worm treatment** – See recipe

- **Prevention** – prevent worm infestation by watching your hygiene. Wash hands with soap after the toilet, before eating and before preparing foods. If you have no soap use soapwort or wood ash.

- **Pawpaw** – Using the white latex from the green fruit take it as follows.

    Young children – 1 teaspoon
    Teens – 2 teaspoon
    Adults – 4 teaspoons

    Take it once on an empty stomach.
    Use Vaseline around the lips first as it is very sticky.
    Drink water afterwards.

Worm Treatment Recipe

Make a mixture of the following:-

1 cup of Wormwood leaves

1 cup of Common Dock *(Rumex lanceolatus)* root

1 cup of chopped Garlic

Mix this all together and take 1 teaspoon of the mixture 3 x day for 5 days

Wound Care

- **Cleaning wounds** – use salt water every two hours if it is a shallow wound or use the antiseptic wash – See recipe

- **Bleeding wounds** – Use chopped yarrow leaves and pack it into the wound and bandage. We had a dog that cut herself really badly around the throat and this was the only thing that would stop the bleeding. We lived 90 minutes away from a vet.

- **Nasturtium** – Macerated nasturtium leaves made into a paste and placed over a septic or dirty wound will clean it.
  Change the dressing daily.
  When clean then use the herbal Antibiotic Ointment as a daily dressing.

- **Yarrow** – Use yarrow Cream – See recipe (Use this for skin grazes and scrapes)

Yarrow Cream

Use for Hemorrhoids, Scratches, Grazes, Varicose Veins.

I have used this myself and for my family. It works very well.

Use a double boiler and add all these ingredients together: -

- 1 cup good aqueous cream
- 1 cup fresh yarrow leaves
- 1 Tblsp thinly grated lemon rind
- 1 Tblsp Eucalyptus leaf powder

Stir for 20 minutes slowly or until liquid.

Cool for 10 minutes and strain.

Add 2 tsp Vitamin E oil and mix gently.

Store in wide mouthed jars in a cool place.

HERBS & THEIR USES

The herbs we use have a variety of functions and healing capabilities. The following list is of the main herbs that we use at our Clinic in Doma, Zimbabwe:

Aloe *(Aloe vera/forex)* –

Beware of taking Aloe Vera internally if there is any sign of rectal bleeding. Rather get the bleeding checked out with a doctor first

- **Rashes, Eczema, Psoriasis** - Open up the leaf and put the clear gel onto the affected area. Rub on the skin three times a day. This has a cooling effect which helps with the irritation.

- **Burns** – open up the leaf and bandage the gel part to the burn – change daily.

- **Constipation** – This is an effective and quick remedy for constipation. Take half cup of the sap daily with plenty of fluid.

- **Haemorrhoids** – Apply topically but can also be taken internally. Half cups of aloe juice three times a day until the haemorrhoid flare up is gone.

- **Ulcers (Peptic ulcers)** – Can be soothed by taking Aloe Vera internally. At the same time the root cause of the ulcer must be dealt with as well e.g. Stress, anxiety.

- **Herpes (shingles)** – Aloe gel applied three times a day with soothe the burning sensation and itchiness.

Basil *(Ocymum basilicum)* –

- **Oral thrush, mouth infections -** Can be used as a mouthwash and gargle. Use one teaspoon of chopped basil in a cup of boiling water. Use every 2 hours.

- **Antibiotic Ointment -** Mix chopped basil with tea tree oil and Vaseline to make an antibiotic ointment. See recipe

- **Insect stings and bites** – A crushed leaf applied to the area will relieve the pain from a sting or bite of an insect.

- **Headaches** – fresh Basil leaves rubbed on the temples for relief of a headache.

- **Nausea** – Taken as a mild tea will relieve nausea.

- **Digestive problems** – Adding fresh Basil leaves to salads and sauces will help digestion.

- **Sore feet and ankles** – fresh basil leaves rubbed around heels and feet or a handful of chopped leaves in two litres of boiling water and left to cool before soaking the feet in will help tired and aching feet. Add lemon grass to the mixture will also freshen your feet.

Blackjack *(Bidens pilosa) –*

- **Indigestion** – Use one teaspoon of the chopped plant to a cup of boiling water as a tea. Use honey to taste. You can have this three times a day.

- **Rheumatism** – Chew the young leaves to relieve rheumatism.

- **Sore eyes** – Make a solution by chopping three fresh clean leaves and mixing with a pinch of salt and 100ml boiled clean water. Use two drops three times a day but keep the solution in the fridge. Make a new solution every day.

Bulbinella *(Bulbine frutescens)* –

- **Rashes, Eczema, Psoriasis** – Squeeze the juice from the leaves onto the skin three times a day. This will stop the irritation instantly.

- **Burns** – open up the leaf and bandage the gel part to the burn – change daily.

- **Insect Bites** – This is an effective and quick remedy for insect bites. Squeeze the juice from the leaf onto the bite or sting.

- **Herpes (shingles)** – Bulbinella juice applied three times a day with soothe the burning sensation and itchiness.

Chickweed *(Stellaria media)* –

- **Rashes, Eczema, Psoriasis** – Chop the leaves and use a cupful of fresh leaves in 500ml of boiling water. Soak for 20 minutes until the liquid is cool. Strain and use as a wash. Wash the area three times a day and let the liquid dry on the area. Use the herbal Ointment afterwards (see recipe)

- **Haemorrhoids** – Crush and macerate the leaf. Use it on Haemorrhoids. It will help relieve some of the swelling and irritation.

- **Indigestion** – Use one teaspoon of the chopped plant to a cup of boiling water as a tea. Use honey to taste. You can have this three times a day.

- **Abscess and boils** – Macerated Chickweed put over a boil or abscess with a dressing will bring the boil or abscess to a head.

Dill *(Anethum graveolens)* -

- **Colic** – In babies use half a tsp powder or freshly chopped Dill in 200ml boiling water. Give a tsp of the mixture three times a day.

- **Stomach pains** – Take one teaspoon three times a day.

- **Digestive problems** – Take as above

- **Breast feeding** – Take to improve milk in nursing mothers. Take one teaspoon three times a day as a tea. Add sugar or honey to taste.
  In addition to this make sure you drink plenty of water.

Feverfew *(Tanacetum parthenium)* –

- **General tonic** – Taken as a tea daily for a "pick me up". Use ½ teaspoon of dried or fresh leaves in a cup of boiling water. Use honey to taste.

- **Migraines** – Use three big leaves to one cup of boiling water. Take this three times a day. (clear this with your doctor first as people have different reasons for migraines)

- **Arthritis** – Use three big leaves to one cup of boiling water. Take this three times a day.

- **Tooth extraction** – Use as a mouthwash.
  Add one cup boiling water to quarter cup chopped leaves. Use three times a day.

- **Constipation** – Use ½ a teaspoon of fresh or dry leaves to one cup of boiling water. Take this three times a day. Remember to drink plenty of water as well.

- **Fever** – Use ½ teaspoon of fresh or dry leaves to one cup of boiling water. Take this three times a day.

- **Woman's problems (female infertility, amenorrhea)** – Place one large cupful of dried leaves in a pot with a lid (shouldn't be a metal pot but an enamel one would be better) and add two cups of warm water.
Bring to the point where it is starting to simmer. Leave to cool overnight.
Strain and use.
Don't keep it for longer than two days and keep it in the refrigerator.
Take a cupful three times a day for three days at a time. Take a break then do it again after five days.

- **Fly repellent** – Feverfew flowers in the kitchen acts as a fly repellent. They will help keep the flies away.

Garlic *(Allium sativum)* –

<u>Remember to clear this with your doctor before using any herb as it may not compliment the drugs you are taking at the time.</u>

<u>If you are allergic to sulphur you need to be careful of garlic as it does have sulphur content.</u>

- **Bronchitis & Catarrh** – Swallow garlic cloves if possible. Take one, three times a day for seven days. If you find it difficult to swallow then use crushed garlic in your food. Eating parsley will help neutralize breath smelling of garlic.

- **High blood pressure** – Use daily in your diet.

- **High cholesterol** - Use regularly in your diet.

- **Chest pains and palpitations** – Take one clove twice a day along with ½ tsp of the Wild Willow leaf or root powder or ½ tablet of Aspirin.

- **Mild infections** – Instead of using antibiotics for mild infections you can also use garlic. Taken over a period of seven to ten days. Remember to clear this with your doctor before using it.

- **Warts** – Crushed garlic placed over a wart and covered with a plaster will irritate the wart and it will fall off. **Warning – On sensitive skin the garlic will burn so be careful.**

Ginger *(Zingiber officinalis)* –

Fresh ginger is always the best way to take ginger but may not be possible. Growing your own in a pot and taking each piece as you need it. It can stay in the pots for years and will keep you supplied with fresh ginger.

- **Stomach pains –**
  Adults - Give half tsp of the powder three times a day as a tea.
  Children - Pinch, as a tea twice a day. Add sugar or honey to taste.

- **Nausea** – use as for stomach pains

- **Flu, Coughs and colds** – use as for stomach pains

- **Travel sickness** – Take one level teaspoon of ginger powder half an hour before travelling. Make sure this is fresh ginger powder and not old as it would have lost most of its properties.

- **Worms** – Hookworms can be cured by taking a dessertspoon of fresh ginger three times a day. For children make the dose much less.

- **Morning sickness** – Taken as a tea and sweetened with honey or brown sugar. Take only half a teaspoon as much as three times a day. Drink this slowly while breathing in the aroma.

Lavender *(Lavandula spica)* –

- **Embrocation** - Can be used for sore muscles, period pains and any aches and pains.
  See the embrocation notes for the recipe.

- **Insomnia** – Take one teaspoon of lavender leaves in a cup of hot water as a tea. Add honey or sugar if needed. For children use much less.

- **Headaches and exhaustion** – Use lavender as a tea to relieve headaches and exhaustion. One teaspoon in a cup of boiling water. Breathing in the aroma at the same time as sipping the tea helps.

- **Mouthwash** – Lavender tea makes an excellent mouthwash for a energy boost when feeling tired and listless.

Lemon Grass *(Cymbopogon citratus)* –

- **Stress** – Lemon grass tea has a calming effect. Use one teaspoon of chopped leaves in a cup of boiling water. Add honey to taste.

- **Insomnia** – Make a tea from Lemon Grass in the evening half an hour before going to bed will help with sleeplessness.

- **Digestion** – Help stimulate digestion. Use it as a tea half an hour before a meal.

- **Flu and colds** – Boil a heaped tablespoon of chopped fresh leaves in one litre of water and use as a steam inhalation three times a day.
  Also drinking it as a tea will also help the cold or flu.

- **Fever** – Add two tablespoons of chopped leaves to two litres boiling water. Drink it warm throughout the day. Make another infusion for the next day and let it soak overnight. Continue for three days. If the fever lasts longer than three days you need to see a doctor.

- **Toothache or bad breath** – Chew fresh washed leaves many times a day.

- **Oils** – You can make a calming oil for baby: -

  Half a cup of chopped and macerated fresh lemon grass leaves soaked in four cups of sunflower oil

with a tablespoon of vitamin E oil added if possible.
Use a glass bottle and leave it to sit in sunshine for up to two weeks.
Don't fill the bottle to the top with oil as it will ferment a little and it will leak out the top.
Strain and use daily for baby.
It has a soothing and calming effect.

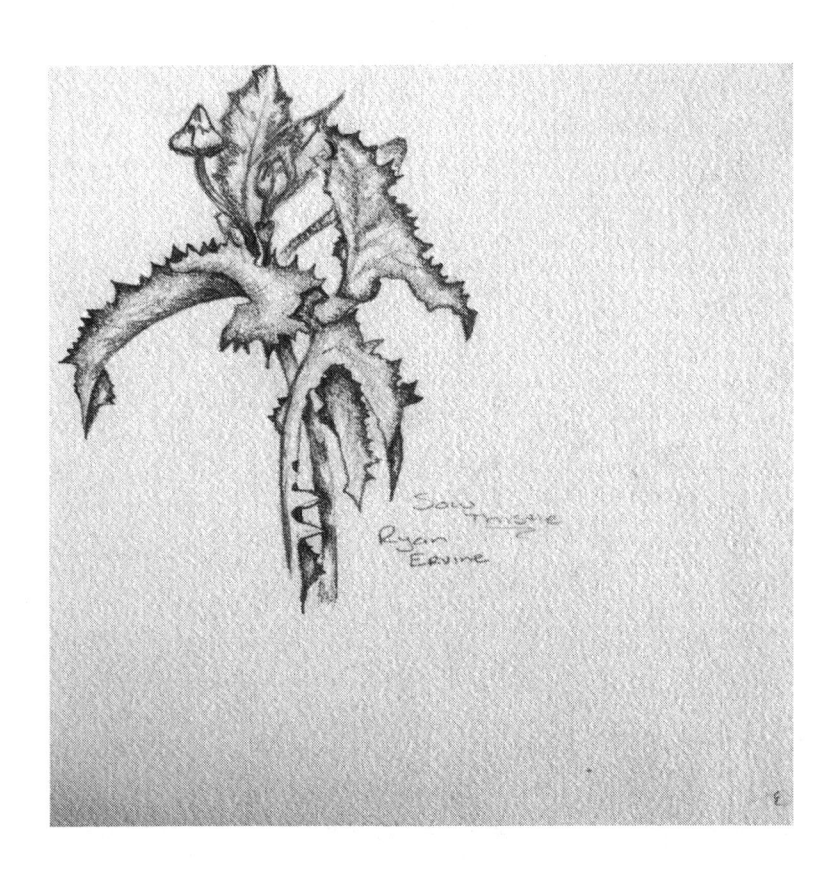

__Marjoram or Oregano__ *(Origanum vulgare)* -

- **Asthma** – Take one tsp three times a day as a tea.

- **Sore throat** - Chew a sprig to relieve a sore throat.

- **Colds, Headaches and stomach disorders** – Pour a cup of boiling water over a quarter cup chopped leaves, flowers and stems.
  This will also relieve coughing.
  Use a quarter of a cup of fresh leaves in a mug of boiling water.

- **Toothache** - Chew a leaf to relieve toothache.

- **Bad breath** – Chewing a leaf will make breath fresher but dental hygiene is important too so find out why halitosis is a problem.

- **Ear wax** – A couple of drops of a warm tea infusion will help to soften wax in the ears.
  Mix one teaspoon of fresh leaves to half a cup of boiling water. Boil for five minutes and cool before using.

- **Bedwetting** – Has been used for bedwetting in older children. Taken as a tea three times a day, last drink at 4pm. Use half a teaspoon.

Mint *(Mentha)* –

There are so many varieties of mint that most of us have one or the other in the garden.

- **Indigestion, Nausea** – Chewing a leaf helps indigestion or as a tea taken at the end of a large meal will help digestion.

- **Flu, Colds** – Use Mint as a steam inhalation. Also take it as a tea to help relieve symptoms. One teaspoon of fresh mint in a cup of boiling water and sweetened with honey will help you feel better.

- **Fly repellent** - Hanging branches of fresh mint in the kitchen is used to keep the flies away. Renew them when they dry out.

- **Headaches** – Taken as a tea will help relieve a headache. Use one teaspoon of fresh mint to a cup of boiling water and sweetened with honey.

- **Vomiting** – Used along with Rooibos as a tea it is very good in small doses taken often during the day.

Moringa _(Moringa oleifera)_ –

Called the **Miracle Tree** because of its many uses and also called the drumstick tree because of the shape of its seed pods.

- **Leaves** - Use as a multi mineral and multi vitamin. Mix dried leaves in the porridge or relish three times a day. Green leaves can be steamed as a vegetable and I also fresh green leaves in a salad.
The Moringa leaves contain these minerals and vitamins:-
    - ✓ Iron
    - ✓ Calcium
    - ✓ Vitamins A, B & C
    - ✓ Phosphorous
    - ✓ Protein

    The leaves are used to combat malnutrition especially amongst children.

    Crushed leaves as a powder and added to food is an appetite stimulant. Also used as a multi vitamin and multi mineral, especially for people with HIV/AIDS, malnutrition and a compressed immune system from parasites.

- **Pods** – When green they can be cooked by cutting into short pieces and cooked and eaten like green beans. They are spicy when young and eaten raw.

- **Seeds** – Crushed seeds sprinkled in dirty water can drop all solids to the bottom and clean the water for use.
  Fry the seeds in oil and can be eaten as nuts.
  Cattle fodder and used as seed cake after extracting the oil.
  Oil used for cosmetics, lamps, cooking.
  A paste made from the seeds is supposed to cure skin infections

- **Roots** – Root bark has some medicinal value. The root bark can be used as a general tonic, laxative, diuretic, enrich the blood, but research on the root bark is ongoing.

Nasturtium *(Tropaeolum majus)* –

Nasturtium is one of the most useful herbs. All parts of the nasturtium can be eaten.

- **Urinary Tract infections, Cystitis, Kidney inflammation** – Infuse one tsp of fresh leaves in 100ml boiling water. Leave to cool, strain and divide the mixture into four sections. Drink one section four times a day.

- **Sore throats** – Chew one medium sized leaf every half an hour. Combine this with half hourly warm salt gargles every 2 hours. I heaped tsp salt to cup warm water. The leaves are very high in vitamin C and also have slight antibiotic tendencies. This does burn a bit so you can't use this for young children.

- **Abscesses, Boils and Dirty wounds** – macerated nasturtium leaves placed over a dirty wound or an open boil will draw out all the dirt and poisons in the wound. Make sure you put Vaseline around the area so that it does not burn the clean skin. Seal off with a closed plaster and change daily until the area is clean. After the area is clean then use the herbal ointment daily until healed with a dressing.

- **Bronchitis and coughing** – Make an tea by using a quarter cup of chopped leaves in a cup of boiling water. Leave for a while, strain and drink three times a day.

- **Because they are high in Vitamin C** and have natural healing properties include them in your salads. The flowers can also be used.

- **Digestive complaints** – A teaspoon of nasturtium seeds, ground and given in half a cup of water four times a day will help digestive problems.

- **Worms** – Use the green seeds.
  Adults can take up to twelve seeds, children up to five seeds, and eat them first thing in the morning on an empty stomach for five days in a row. They do burn a bit so for very young children you won't be able to do this.

Neem *(Azadirachta indica)* -

General

- **Cuts**: - Use as a wash and an ointment. Can also use it internally.

- **Burns**: - As an ointment made with the seed oil.

- **Sprain and Bruises**: - Neem tea, Crushed leaves and bandaged, Neem oil and leaf extract

- **Earache**: - 1 clove garlic, 1 tsp vegetable oil, 2 drops camphor oil, 5 drops Neem leaf extract. Use this as drops 3 x day.

- **Fever**: - Make a Neem tea (5 leaves). Repeat 4 hrly.

- **Sore throat**: - Make a mouthwash and gargle – use the tea recipe 4-6hrly.

- **TB**: - Take a Neem tea several times a day. Also do Neem steam inhalations 4 x day.

- **Food Poisoning**: - Take a cup of Neem tea 6 times a day.

Viral Infections

- **Chicken pox**: - Make a paste from the Neem leaves and rub onto skin. Bathing in Neem tea, Neem tea taken internally, Adults can eat leaves 4 times a day.

- **Herpes Zoster**: - Take internally during stressful periods. Use Neem cream and leaf poultice on the blisters.

- **Colds**: - Drink mild Neem tea twice a week as a preventative. To treat, drink mild Neem tea 3 x day.

- **Hepatitis**: - Drinking Neem tea regularly can protect the liver.

Fungal Infections

- **Ringworm**: - Make a paste from the fresh leaves mixed with the seed oil. Place over the area and change daily.

- **Jock itch**: - Dry the Neem leaves and mix with baby powder on a one to one basis. Use this three times a day.

- **Athletes Foot**: - Corn Starch powder with powdered Neem leaves. As a preventative. If infected already then macerate one cup of fresh Neem leaves and add to 500ml of boiling water. When cool enough soak your feet for 10 minutes three times a day.

- ❖ **Yeast Infections**: -
  Vaginal – Neem based cream and to douche with a Neem infusion. 1 tsp Neem to a cup of boiling water.
  Penile – Use a Neem based cream 4 x day.
  Oral – Drink Neem tea along with other treatments to heal internally.

- ❖ **Oral Thrush**: - Neem tea taken internally and as a mouthwash 3 x day.

Sexually Transmitted Diseases

- ❖ **Gonorrhea, Syphilis, Vaginal Infections**: - Take Neem leaf tea 4 x day. Bathe in water with Neem oil

Skin Infections

- ❖ **Psoriasis, Eczema, Vitiligo, Acne, Dry skin, Skin Ulcers, Itchy scalp, Rashes, Dandruff**: - Use a Neem tea to bathe with and let the juice dry on the skin. Then use a Neem cream. Neem shampoo will help with itchy scalp and dandruff. Use the Neem oil or extract in baths for itchy and dry skin along with a Neem based cream.

Periodontal

- ❖ **Toothache**: - Drops of leaf extract & 1 clove near the pain.

- ❖ **Bleeding Gums**: - Use Neem tea as a mouthwash

Circulatory

- **Hypertension**:- Drink Neem tea 3 x day.

- **High Cholesterol**:- Take Neem tea daily for a month at a time.

Neem Cream

To make Neem cream mix the following: -

1 Cup dry Neem leaves

1 Cup Aqueous Cream

1 Tablespoon grated lemon rind

Stir this over a low heat or a double boiler until the aqueous cream is liquefied. Cool slightly and strain.

When cool add 2 teaspoons of vitamin E Oil.

Store in a wide mouthed glass jar in a cool place.

To make an ointment exchange the aqueous cream for Petroleum Jelly.

Parsley *(Petroselinum crispum)* –

Please don't stop any medications you are on and consult your doctor about using herbs.

- **Diuretic** – helps to reduce swollen legs etc (gets rid of excess water in the body)

- **Kidney & Bladder infections** – Pour a cup of boiling water over a teaspoon of chopped parsley leaves. Leave to stand for five minutes and then drink. Also chew parsley daily. Drink this mixture three times a day for seven days. Take a three day break and then continue.

- **Weaning infants** – Fresh parsley worn inside the bra against the nipple will dry up the breast milk.

- **Arthritis, Sore joints, and anaemia** – make a strong tea. A handful of leaves to two cups of boiling water. Cool, strain and drink twice daily.

- **Halitosis** – For people who have been eating garlic or onions. Chewing fresh parsley can help freshen your breath.

- **Cancer** – Including fresh parsley in your daily salads is now being looked at as a preventative measure as it is packed with vitamins and minerals.

- **Diabetes** – Taken as a strong tea like for bladder infections is supposed to help balance sugar levels.

Rocket *(Eruca vesicaria)* -

- **Cleanser** – This helps to rid the body of pollutants. Add to diet regularly as a fresh salad herb.

- **Coughs** – A tablespoon boiled with a tablespoon of honey and a tablespoon of water to make a cough syrup. Take the cough syrup three times a day. Adults will use one dessert spoon and children half.

- **Swollen legs** – Can be used instead of parsley as a diuretic. Use in vegetable dishes and salads. Take it daily if you can.

- **Malnutrition, bleeding gums, as a Vitamin, Bladder ailments** – Include regularly (daily) in diet. Fresh rocket must be eaten in salads daily.

Rosemary *(Rosmarinus officinalis)* -

- **Blood pressure abnormalities** – Take half a teaspoon three times a day as a tea. Sweeten with honey or sugar if you need to.

- **Headache** - Especially for children under 15 as they cannot take aspirin. Make a solution of one heaped teaspoon of rosemary to a cup of boiling water.

    Children 3 – 6yrs – ¼ (quarter) tsp 3 x day
    7yrs – 12 yrs – ½ (half) tsp 3 x day
    Teens and adults – 1 tsp 3 x day

Remember that headaches are usually caused from not drinking enough water.

- **Convalescent's tonic** – This is really good for people recovering from illness. Make a tea from mixing a quarter cup of fresh rosemary with a cup of boiling water. Sweeten to taste with honey if needed. Take twice a day.

- **Arthritis** – Using fresh rosemary in salads and cooking can help alleviate the symptoms of arthritis.

Rue *(Ruta graveolens)* –

Can be toxic so be careful (Can cause liver damage)

- **Epilepsy** – Indigenous people in Africa have used this for epilepsy for generations. We have had some good results with this treatment as many people cannot buy the tablets they need to control their epilepsy.
  Mix one teaspoon freshly chopped rue leaves in 500ml boiling water. Strain and allow to cool. Take one teaspoon of the solution three times a day for epilepsy.
  Don't just stop the prescription tablets the person is on, they must be weaned slowly onto the Rue treatment. The treatment may depend on what has cause the epilepsy in the first place. Please check with your doctor first as this could be dangerous if not monitored properly.

- **Breast pains** - Fresh Rue leaves rubbed on a breast and the above mixture used for five days can help breast pains in woman and sometimes woman who may have benign lumps in their breasts.

- **Toothache** – Local people use a rolled up leaf in the hole in the tooth for toothache.

- **Earache** – Roll a fresh leaf and place in the entrance to the ear. Don't force it in.
- **Boils & Abscesses** – A lotion on a dressing covering the area will draw the abscess.
  Make a brew of one teaspoon chopped leaves in 500 ml boiling water.

Leave to soak and cool for 20 minutes. Soak the dressing in this before placing and binding over the area.
Change it twice a day.

- **Lice, Skin Parasites** – Use a wash mixed as above to get rid of the parasites.
  Repeat daily for three days.
  Use this along with the other hygiene factors listed under the Scabies heading.

Soapwort *(Saponaria officinalis)* –

- **Wound wash** – This herb contains sapiens so can be cut up and crushed then mixed with water as a body wash or wound wash.

- **Rashes** – as above but let the juice dry on the skin then use the herbal antibiotic ointment. Do this twice a day.

- **Psoriasis** – You can use the stems, leaves and flowers. Remember the root must not be taken internally as it is known to be poisonous. Boil two cups of fresh leaves with two litres of water for fifteen minutes. Cool, strain and use as a lotion three times a day.

- **Eczema** – Can use it the same as above. Leave to dry on the affected areas.

Sour fig *(Carpobrotus edulis)* –

The fruit and juice from the leaves of this plant have been used by indigenous people for years. They contain antiseptic properties.

- **Extraction** – Use the fleshy leaves and pound them first with a mortar and pestle (glass or ceramic) then strained in a sieve overnight.

- **Sore throat** – Chew a leaf tip or make a mixture as follows: -
  1 part vinegar
  1 part honey
  1 part sour fig leaf juice.
  1 part Lemon Juice
  Take a tablespoon three times a day.

- **Mouth infections** – Chew a leaf many times through the day.

- **Burns** - Smothering the burn in the juice and dressing straight away. This works the same as Aloe Vera gel.

- **Skin rashes** – Juice from the leaves rubbed onto the skin three times a day and left to dry on the skin.

- **Indigestion, Diarrhoea** – Take a dessertspoon full of the juice three times a day. This works the same way as Aloe Vera.

Sweet Violet *(Viola odorata)* -

- **Headaches** - Flowers and leaves can be chewed to relieve headaches. Chew three leaves twice a day.

- **Laxative** – (for constipation) make a tea by adding quarter teaspoon of chopped leaves and flowers to a cup of boiling water. Add honey to taste. You can take this three times a day. Drink plenty of clean water in between.

- **Flu, colds, mucus,** - Make a tea by adding a cup of boiling water to quarter cup of chopped leaves and flowers. Stand for a while and then drink.

- **Eczema & Rashes** – make a strong tea and use as a wash twice a day. This soothes the itching and irritation.

- **Painful uterus (lower abdomen pains)** - Take one teaspoon three times a day of dried violet leaves and flowers.

- **Cancer** – Chew violet leaves and you can also use crushed leaves as a poultice for skin cancer and growths.

Sweet wormwood *(Artemisia affra)* –

- **Diarrhoea and stomach pains** – making a tea with half a teaspoon of fresh or dried leaves in a cup of boiling water.
  Use honey to taste as this can be very bitter.
  Adults – 1 tsp 3 x day.
  Children – ¼ (quarter) tsp 3 x day.
  Babies – **don't give.**

- **Worms** – This can work as a vermifuge and has been used by the indigenous people in parts of Zimbabwe as it grows wild in some areas.
  Adults – 1 tsp 3 x day for 4 days.
  Children – ¼ (quarter) tsp 3 x day for 4 days.
  Babies **– Do not use.**

- **Colds, whooping Cough –** My grandmother used to use this as it grew wild in the hills where she lived. Taken as a tea three times a day. Use the same dosage as for diarrhoea. Sweeten with honey.

- **Earache and ear infections –** Make a brew with two tablespoons of fresh leaves and add this to half litre (500ml) boiling water.
  Sweeten with fresh honey and take two teaspoons morning and night for four days. Don't exceed the four days.

To make ear drops – Use one teaspoon leaves in a cup of boiling water. Cool and drop two drops into the ear, three times a day to relieve earache.

- **Coughs** – A cough mixture can be made with Sweet Wormwood, Brown Sugar or Honey, Thyme, Ginger, Rosemary and Mint.
Use one part of each and one part water.
Heat up together until nearly boiling.
Leave to cool, strain and place the liquid in a fridge. You can add Brandy (Alcohol) to this as well which will preserve the shelf life but keeping it in the fridge will work without the brandy.

- **Headaches** – You can cure a headache by putting a rolled up leaf in the nostrils.
The aroma will relieve a headache.

- **Bronchitis & Respiratory infections** – Use a handful in boiling water as a steam inhalation.

Tansy *(Tanacetum vulgare)* -

Be very careful of this herb. It can be toxic if not given correctly. We only use this if we need to.

- **Fevers** – One tsp chopped leaves to 250ml boiling water.
  Adults – 1 tsp 3 x day.
  Children and babies don't use. Rather use Yarrow.
  Don't give more than advised as it can be toxic.

- **Kidney problems** – 1 teaspoon three times a day as a tea with plenty of water.

- **Jaundice** – 1 teaspoon three times a day as a tea with plenty of water.

- **Reduces high blood pressure** – 1 teaspoon three times a day as a tea with plenty of water.

- **Mouth infections** – Use as a gargle. Half a teaspoon of fresh leaves to a mug of boiling water.

- **Worms** – Use half a tsp of fresh chopped leaves two times a day in adults. **Don't use for children.**

- **Insecticide** – Hang bunches of leaves in the kitchen to keep flies away.

Tea Tree *(Melaleuca alternifolia)* -

Tea tree oil must NOT be taken internally in any situations as it is extremely toxic

Tea tree is a tree native to Australia. Used traditionally for years by the local aborigines.

- **Fungicide – Ringworm, Athletes foot, Jock itch.** Use mixed with Vaseline as an ointment. Use three times a day.

- **Anti Viral – Shingles, Cold sores, Chicken Pox, measles.** Use mixed with Vaseline as an ointment and use three times a day.

- **Inhalation therapies – Bronchitis, Asthma, Flu, Hay fever, Whooping Cough.** Drops in a basin of boiling water.

- **Thrush - vaginal and Oral** – Use added to warm water as a vaginal douche or neat on a cotton bud for oral but **use with extreme caution and not in small babies.**

- **Abscess** – added to hot water as a compress for **drawing boils, abscesses** – use every 2 hrs

- **Skin conditions – Acne, Eczema, Scabies** . Use as an ointment or add a few drops to warm water as a daily wash

- **Bites and Stings, Burns, Wounds**. Make a lotion and use as a daily wash or to dab on hourly if for bites and stings.

- **Earache – use with caution.** A couple of drops to 10ml of warm water and use 3 drops into the ear three times a day. **Don't use if eardrum is perforated.**

- **Gingivitis** – As a mouthwash added to warm water but must **not** be swallowed. Use three times a day – 3 drops to half a cup of water.

- **Warts** – Make an ointment using crushed aspirin and tea tree oil – 300g Vaseline, 80 drops tea tree oil, 5 heaped teaspoons crushed aspirin, put on three times a day.

- **Tonsillitis, Sore throats** – A couple of drops added to warm water and used as a gargle – **Must NOT be swallowed**

Thyme *(Thymus vulgaris)* –

- **HIV/Aids** – Loss of weight in HIV/AIDS patients Adults – Take one teaspoon three times a day as a tea. Sweeten with honey if needed.

- **Oral thrush** – as above. This works for Candida infections throughout the body.

- **Flu, colds and coughs** – Take half tsp in a cup of boiling water as a tea three times a day and sweeten with honey.
  The lemon scented thyme is a good one to use for this.

- **Calmative** – Can be used as a tea for stress.

Yarrow *(Achillea millefolium)* –

- **Fever** - in children and adults –
    Babies 1yr onwards – ¼ (quarter) tsp 3 x day.
    Children - ½ (half) tsp 3 x day
    Adults – 1 tsp 3 x day.

- **Toothache** – put a piece of the leaf in the hole in the tooth as a temporary measure to help the pain or chew the leaf on the tooth that is paining you.

- **Bleeding** – Chopped yarrow put over the wound & bandaged in place will stop the bleeding quickly. I had to use this treatment for one of our dogs once who had an accident and it worked really well.

- **Menstrual bleeding** - Mix equal parts dried yarrow with equal parts dry parsley
    Use one teaspoon of this mixture three times a day for excessive menstrual bleeding.
    Take as a tea.

- **Earache** – Make a yarrow brew – One teaspoon of fresh Yarrow leaves in half a cup of boiling water. Strain and Cool. Drop two drops into the ear three times a day. **(Only use this if there is no pus present. If pus is present then you must see your doctor)**

- **Cramps** – An infusion of flowers taken through the day will help cramp. Take half a teaspoon of flowers in a cup of boiling water as a tea.

- **Diuretic** – The flowers also have diuretic properties and can be taken as a tea throughout the day. Dosage is same as above.

- **Colds & Flu** – Taken as a tea during the day will help symptoms of flu and reduce fever. Also using yarrow along with lavender, rosemary, mint and lemon grass leaves in boiling water as a steam inhalation will help clear sinuses.

CLINIC INTERNSHIPS & TRAINING

We routinely train people in herbal medicine at our Clinic in Doma, Zimbabwe. If you have an interest in learning about herbal medicine and bush medicine, please contact Judy Ervine at ervestpl@mweb.co.zw to make arrangements.

OUR BASIC NEEDS

We do have basic needs that are the base of our ointments and oils that we use. We count on donations from faithful supporters to meet our needs.

Vaseline. We will use a drum (175kg) every 3 months, to make the ointments that we use in the clinic.

Vinegar, (Brown vinegar and Apple Cider Vinegar).

Oils (Eucalyptus, Camphorated, Tea tree oil, Clove oil, cooking oil)

Spice powders (Cayenne pepper or Piri piri pepper – We do grown some of our own but also run out occasionally during the winter months.

Herbs – Garlic and Ginger (we do try and grow our own or get from local people who have grown but often we run out during the winter months)

Equipment – Gloves, Masks, Surgical Blades, Dressings & Bandages (conforming & crepe)

Donations for the Clinic can be made to:

Eden Ministries
2133 Berkey Avenue
Goshen, Indiana, USA 46526

Your donations save lives!

OUR DREAM

Future Goals.

1. Our first goal is to have a slightly bigger clinic with a counseling room and an isolated room for the dressings and the washing area. Sometimes the wounds are very septic and the smell so bad that we have to close the entire clinic and work outside, so it would be better to isolate that section with an extractor fan. Although often during a clinic day there is no power for fans and so with the heat it can be difficult. We would also like to have a cottage built onto this clinic for our resident health worker who often has to put people up at night because they have come from so far away and to join that to a four bed ward where we can have people sleep over and be monitored if need be.
Costing for this we have worked on around US$ 8000.00 (prices can change)

2. Our next goal is to have a mobile clinic running so we can reach people in the very remote areas. We sometimes have people walking for two days and sleeping in the bush by the side of the road on the way, to try and reach us for medical

help. This would also combine with teaching health workers in far reaching areas about basic herbal medicines for basic medical needs i.e. – Diarrhea, Scabies, Flu, cuts and wounds. Also to combine this with teaching about nutrition and hygiene. Our idea is a four wheel drive vehicle and an off road trailer as we would need to stay overnight in the field. We have looked into a Toyota Land Cruiser with a closed van back and an off road trailer which is equipped with water storage, cooking facility and a tent cover.

Prices we saw for these were –

Toyota L Cruiser – Around U$60 000.00 (good second hand – 40 – 45 000)

Trailer – Off road (fully equipped) – Around U$10 000.00

3. We also want to join our seed program with the mobile clinic and to start teaching people on the right foods to grow by supplying their first seeds and monitoring the growing seasons. This has been done before but we have not had the ability to follow up and monitor closely. This would have to be done with one settlement area at a time concentrating on one person and then they would be able to teach the others in the settlement.

However this takes a lot of time and it's the old saying.

Give a person a fish

and they will have a meal

Teach them how to fish

and they will have a lifetime of meals.

ABOUT THE AUTHOR

Judy Ervine is a State Registered Nurse and a Registered Herbal Practitioner who operates the Eden Herbal Medical Clinic in Doma, Zimbabwe. She has treated more than 21,000 destitute people at the Clinic at no charge. Her herbal knowledge is considerable, and she is a gifted medical practitioner. She and her husband Rory have three sons: Sean, Craig and Ryan. All three boys are professional cricketers. Judy is also an accomplished watercolorist and artist. She is a passionate and compassionate follower of Jesus Christ, using her many gifts for His Kingdom.

Made in the USA
Middletown, DE
22 March 2015